Fast Facts

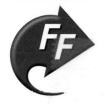

Fast Facts:
Celiac Disease

Second edition

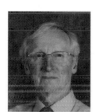

Geoffrey Holmes MD PhD FRCP
Consultant Physician and Gastroenterologist
Royal Derby Hospital
Derby, UK

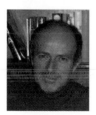

Carlo Catassi MD
Associate Professor, Department of Pediatrics
Università Politecnica delle Marche, Ancona, Italy and
Co Director, Center For Celiac Research
University of Maryland School of Medicine
Baltimore, MD, USA

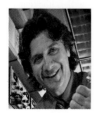

Alessio Fasano MD
Professor of Pediatrics, Medicine and Physiology
Director, Mucosal Biology Research Center
University of Maryland School of Medicine
Baltimore, MD, USA

Declaration of Independence
This book is as balanced and as practical as we can make it.
Ideas for improvement are always welcome: feedback@fastfacts.com

HEALTH PRESS

Fast Facts: Celiac Disease
First published 2000
Second edition August 2009

Health Press Limited, Elizabeth House, Queen Street, Abingdon,
Oxford OX14 3LN, UK
Tel: +44 (0)1235 523233
Fax: +44 (0)1235 523238

Book orders can be placed by telephone or via the website.
For regional distributors or to order via the website, please go to:
www.fastfacts.com
For telephone orders, please call +44 (0)1752 202301 (UK and Europe),
1 800 247 6553 (USA, toll free), +1 419 281 1802 (Americas)
or +61 (0)2 9698 7755 (Asia–Pacific).

Fast Facts is a trademark of Health Press Limited.

The publisher and the authors have made every effort to ensure the accuracy of this
book, but cannot accept responsibility for any errors or omissions.

For all drugs, please consult the product labeling approved in your country for
prescribing information.

A CIP record for this title is available from the British Library.

Cover image is a scanning electron micrograph of the wall of the small intestine in a
patient with celiac disease. The mucosa appears flat and atrophied due to the loss of
villi. Reproduced with permission from Professors PM Motta and FN Magliocca/
Science Photo Library.

ISBN 978-1-905832-56-9

Holmes G (Geoffrey)
Fast Facts: Celiac Disease/
Geoffrey Holmes, Carlo Catassi, Alessio Fasano

Typesetting and page layout by Zed, Oxford, UK.
Printed by Latimer Trend & Company Limited, Plymouth, UK.

Text printed with vegetable inks on biodegradable and recyclable
paper manufactured using elemental chlorine free (ECF) wood
pulp from well managed forests.

FSC
Mixed Sources
Product group from well-managed
forests and other controlled sources
Cert no. SGS-COC-005493
www.fsc.org
© 1996 Forest Stewardship Council

Glossary of abbreviations

AEA: anti-endomysial antibody

AGA: anti-gliadin antibody

Allele: one of the different forms of a gene

Anti-tTG: anti-tissue transglutaminase antibody

ARA: anti-reticulin antibody

CD: cluster of differentiation

CT: computed tomography

DEXA: dual-energy X-ray absorptiometry

DH: dermatitis herpetiformis

EATL: enteropathy-associated T-cell lymphoma

ELISA: enzyme-linked immunosorbent assay

Genotype: the two haplotypes on parental chromosomes

GFD: gluten-free diet

GH: growth hormone

Haplotype: combination of alleles at multiple loci that are transmitted together on the same chromosome

HLA: human leukocyte antigen

IEL: intraepithelial lymphocyte

IFN: interferon

Ig: immunoglobulin

IL: interleukin

Incidence: the number of new cases of a disease in a defined population during a specified period of time

LAD: linear IgA disease

MCV: mean corpuscular volume

MRI: magnetic resonance imaging

NHL: non-Hodgkin lymphoma

PET: positron emission tomography

ppm: parts per million

Prevalence: the total number of cases of a disease present in a defined population at a specified time

SD: standard deviation

TCR: T-cell receptor

TJ: tight junction

TNF: tumor necrosis factor

tTG: tissue transglutaminase

Introduction

The interest in celiac disease is now truly international: the corpus of knowledge about celiac disease is growing exponentially, with contributions from researchers around the world. Important advances have made a new edition of this book necessary. For example, new understandings of the mechanisms responsible for producing damage to the small-intestinal mucosa are leading to potential new treatments that may allow patients to consume gluten products without risk of ill health. There is even talk of preventing celiac disease. The age at which gluten is introduced in the diet in infancy, together with the gluten load and breastfeeding, are factors that determine the onset of the disorder; by manipulating these factors it is hoped to prevent celiac disease from arising.

It is easy to chart the landmarks in our increasing understanding of celiac disease. In 1888, Samuel Gee put celiac disease on the map with his delightful paper *On the celiac affection* in which he described the clinical features in children with remarkable accuracy. He predicted, with prophetic insight, that cure would come from manipulation of the diet. Idiopathic steatorrhea, or non-tropical sprue, was much later recognized to be celiac disease in adults.

The modern era was ushered in when Willem Dicke announced in 1950 that gluten damaged patients with celiac disease. This led to effective treatment with a gluten-free diet (GFD) and provided researchers with a protein to explore by means of newly emerging techniques in biochemistry and immunology. In the mid-1950s, it was possible for the first time to obtain peroral biopsies of the small intestine, so that celiac disease could be defined in morphologic terms. At the beginning of the 1970s, genetic markers of celiac disease were identified. In the 1980s, the ability to take intestinal biopsies using fiber-optic endoscopes and the development of serological tests for celiac disease greatly facilitated diagnosis. A decade later, the first screening studies showed celiac disease to be one of the commonest lifelong disorders in the Western world, causing considerable ill health and increases in mortality.

In the 1960s, an enteropathy was found in patients with dermatitis herpetiformis similar to that in celiac disease, with a rash that was gluten sensitive. Recently, some neurological disorders have also been identified as a manifestation of gluten sensitivity, so-called gluten neuropathy or gluten ataxia. Different forms of transglutaminase appear to determine which organs are affected by gluten. So the spectrum of gluten sensitivity is wider than first thought and may continue to expand.

Celiac disease can now be identified reliably thanks to the refinement of the serum anti-tissue transglutaminase antibody test. This has led to a reappraisal of the diagnostic criteria and has brought into question whether intestinal biopsy is always necessary. The genetic basis for celiac disease is proving difficult to establish, but progress is being made. Knowledge of the susceptibility genes carried by individuals should allow an accurate estimate of the risk they have of developing the condition.

Reassuringly for patients, several recent studies have shown that malignant complications are less common than previously thought. Once developed, however, lymphoma carries a very poor prognosis. One form of refractory celiac disease has been identified as a precursor to lymphoma, and attempts are under way to find a successful treatment that would reduce the malignant risk.

Finally, the effects of a GFD on the quality of life of those with celiac disease have been explored. Legislation regarding gluten-free products that should offer better guidance to patients has recently been enacted in both the USA and the EU.

Despite this remarkable progress the diagnosis of celiac disease is easily overlooked, resulting in a large number of undiagnosed patients who are unwell and exposed to various health risks in the community. The practical challenge for doctors and other healthcare workers is to identify these patients and offer them a GFD that will restore the majority to full health and may prevent the development of complications. This fully updated second edition of *Fast Facts: Celiac Disease* offers a concise account of the condition and explores all of the latest findings in relation to its diagnosis and management, with the hope that it will help to meet this challenge.

Definition

Celiac disease, or gluten-sensitive enteropathy, is characterized by immune-mediated damage to the jejunal mucosa that is triggered in genetically susceptible individuals by gluten, a protein complex in wheat, rye and barley cereals. Definitions of celiac disease have revolved around abnormalities found in the jejunal mucosa as well as responses to gluten withdrawal and challenge and the associated clinical reactions. The finding that certain antibodies are markedly associated with celiac disease has added an important dimension to the definition of the disease.

In practice, the diagnosis is usually straightforward and is based on:
- typical serology of positive anti-endomysial (AEA) and anti-tissue transglutaminase antibodies (anti-tTG)
- characteristic appearance of a small-bowel biopsy
- satisfactory response to a gluten-free diet (GFD).

Furthermore, celiac disease develops in the context of a positive HLA-DQ2 and/or -DQ8 haplotype.

For many years, the mucosal changes in celiac disease have been described as total, subtotal or partial villous atrophy; more recently, in an effort to standardize reporting, the modified Marsh classification has been widely adopted for clinical use (Table 1.1). In this classification, types 3a, 3b and 3c equate to partial, subtotal and total villous atrophy, respectively, and are characteristic of untreated celiac disease. It is clear, however, that the range of gluten sensitivity is wider than previously realized; several forms of celiac disease are now identified, and the modified Marsh classification recognizes a spectrum of mucosal change from a mild to a severe abnormality (Figure 1.1). Factors such as the amount of ingested gluten, gastrointestinal infection or the stress of a pregnancy or operation may influence the gradual shift from a minimal-change enteropathy to the typical flat lesion characteristic of celiac disease.

Typical celiac disease
Typical celiac disease is characterized by the classic features of malabsorption, such as weight loss, chronic diarrhea, steatorrhea and,

TABLE 1.1

Modified Marsh classification of mucosal lesions in celiac disease

Type	IELs/100 enterocytes	Crypts	Villi
0	< 25*	Normal	Normal
1	> 25	Normal	Normal
2	> 25	Hyperplastic	Normal
3a	> 25	Hyperplastic	Mild atrophy
3b	> 25	Hyperplastic	Marked atrophy
3c	> 25	Hyperplastic	Absent

Type 0	Normal mucosa; celiac disease very unlikely
Type 1	Infiltrative lesion; may indicate celiac disease and progress to a type 3 lesion
Type 2	Hyperplastic lesion; may indicate celiac disease
Type 3	Destructive lesion; spectrum of changes characteristic of untreated celiac disease. Patients may be symptomatic or asymptomatic

*The Marsh–Oberhuber classification indicated that 40 IELs/100 enterocytes should be the cut-off point. Based on recent data, the upper limit of the normal range has been reduced to 25 IELs/100 enterocytes.
IEL, intraepithelial lymphocyte.

in infants, failure to thrive. Biopsies from the small intestine usually show types 3a to 3c mucosal lesions but occasionally damage can be less severe.

Atypical celiac disease

Atypical celiac disease is characterized by often isolated, usually extraintestinal, manifestations. These include chronic fatigue, anemia, short stature, pubertal delay, arthralgia and infertility. The degree of small-intestinal damage varies from a type 1 lesion to a fully expressed gluten-sensitive enteropathy (type 3c). Atypical forms are encountered more commonly than typical forms in clinical practice.

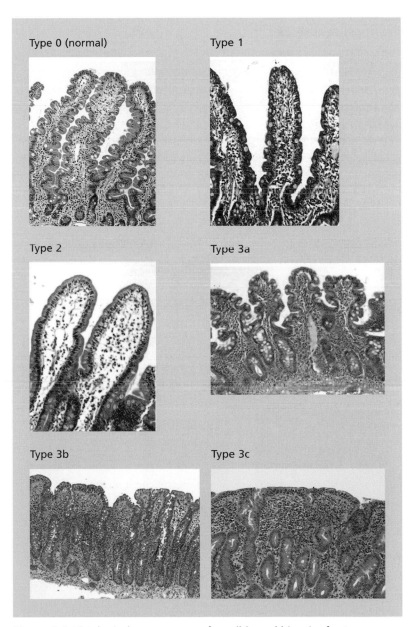

Type 0 (normal) Type 1

Type 2 Type 3a

Type 3b Type 3c

Figure 1.1 Histological appearances of small-bowel biopsies for types 0 to 3c according to the Marsh classification modified by Oberhuber. Reproduced courtesy of I. Bearzi, Department of Pathology, Università Politecnica delle Marche, Ancona, Italy.

Silent celiac disease

Silent celiac disease is occasionally found following serological screening in patients who are asymptomatic. Not uncommonly, some report an improvement in psychophysical wellbeing with a GFD. The degree of small-intestinal damage can vary from a type 1 lesion to a fully expressed gluten-sensitive enteropathy (type 3c).

Potential celiac disease

Potential celiac disease is characterized by a type 1 lesion. Patients are positive for anti-tTG and/or AEA and/or subepithelial deposits of tTG-specific immunoglobulin A in the biopsy (Figure 1.2). They can be well

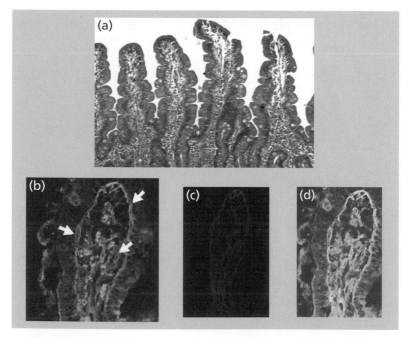

Figure 1.2 Sections of the jejunum from a patient with potential celiac disease, showing (a) a normal villous architecture with hematoxylin and eosin staining; (b) subepithelial immunoglobulin (Ig)A deposits (arrows) and (c) tissue transglutaminase-2 (tTG-2). (d) The yellow color in this composite picture indicates co-localization of IgA deposits and tTG-2. Reproduced from Salmi et al. 2006 with permission of Blackwell Publishing copyright © 2006.

or have intestinal symptoms that may respond to a GFD. In time, they may develop a flat mucosa.

Latent celiac disease

Patients with latent celiac disease have a normal biopsy while on a normal diet, but evidence of a flat or severely damaged mucosa at some other time while on a normal diet that recovers on a GFD.

Key points – definition

- Celiac disease is characterized by immune-mediated damage to the jejunal mucosa that is triggered in genetically susceptible individuals by gluten, a protein complex in wheat, rye and barley.
- The celiac enteropathy ranges from an isolated increase in intraepithelial lymphocytes in apparently normal villi (type 1 lesion) to a flat mucosa showing a type 3c abnormality.
- The clinical spectrum of celiac disease includes typical, atypical, silent, potential and latent forms.

Key references

Corazza GR, Villanacci V. Coeliac disease. *J Clin Pathol* 2005;58: 573–4.

Dickey W, Hughes DF, McMillan SA. Patients with serum IgA endomysial antibodies and intact duodenal villi: clinical characteristics and management options. *Scand J Gastroenterol* 2005;40:1240–3.

Marsh MN. Gluten, major histocompatibility complex, and the small intestine. A molecular and immunobiologic approach to the spectrum of gluten sensitivity ('celiac sprue'). *Gastroenterology* 1992;102:330–54.

Oberhuber G, Granditsch G, Vogelsang H. The histopathology of coeliac disease: time for a standardized report scheme for pathologists. *Eur J Gastroenterol Hepatol* 1999;11:1185–94.

Salmi TT, Collin P, Järvinen O et al. Immunoglobulin A autoantibodies against transglutaminase 2 in the small intestinal mucosa predict forthcoming coeliac disease. *Aliment Pharmacol Ther* 2006;24:541–52.

Thirty years ago, celiac disease was considered to be a rare disorder affecting individuals of European origin, with onset of symptoms during the first few years of life. Diagnosis was based on the recognition of typical gastrointestinal symptoms and confirmed by small-intestinal biopsy. The introduction of highly sensitive and specific serological tests to detect, first, anti-gliadin (AGA) and, later, anti-endomysial (AEA) and anti-tissue transglutaminase antibodies (anti-tTG) showed an unsuspected high frequency of clinically atypical or even silent forms of celiac disease. Using these simple tests as a first-level screening procedure, a large number of studies have shown that celiac disease is one of the commonest lifelong disorders found worldwide (Figure 2.1).

In Europe, where many studies have been carried out, the prevalence of celiac disease mostly ranges between 0.5 and 1% of the general population, with a trend toward higher values (up to 2%) among genetically isolated groups (e.g. in Finland). This prevalence is far

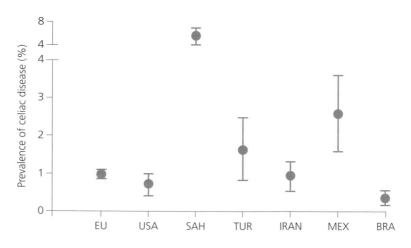

Figure 2.1 Prevalence (and 95% confidence interval) of celiac disease in different countries. BRA, Brazil; EU, Europe; MEX, Mexico; SAH, Western Sahara; TUR, Turkey.

higher than for other permanent conditions, such as familial hypercholesterolemia, selective immunoglobulin A deficiency, type 1 diabetes mellitus and congenital hypothyroidism. Until recently, celiac disease was perceived to be rare in North America. This misconception has been corrected by a large screening study that has shown the prevalence in the US population to be about 1%, the same as in Europe. Similar disease frequencies have been reported from countries mostly populated by individuals of European origin (e.g. Canada, Brazil, Argentina, Australia and New Zealand).

Celiac disease is increasingly reported from areas of the developing world, particularly North Africa, the Middle East and India, where it contributes substantially to childhood morbidity and mortality. In the Saharawis, an Arab population living in Western Sahara, the prevalence is 5.6%. The reasons for this high figure are unclear, but could primarily relate to genetic factors and to the high level of consanguinity in this population. In North India, celiac disease is particularly common in the so-called 'celiac belt', a part of the country where wheat is a staple food. Clinical series from India usually describe typical cases, with chronic diarrhea, anemia and stunting being the commonest symptoms in children (Figure 2.2). However, atypical cases present with short stature, anemia, abdominal distension, rickets, constipation, type 1 diabetes and delayed puberty.

There are only anecdotal reports of celiac disease in other parts of the world (e.g. Sub-Saharan African countries, China, Japan and Central America). The genes predisposing to celiac disease are common throughout the world, however, with few exceptions (e.g. native Highlanders from Papua New Guinea) (Table 2.1). Furthermore, wheat is increasingly being consumed by populations that previously ate other staple cereals such as rice or millet (Figure 2.3). These factors suggest that celiac disease will be reported increasingly from countries that so far have been almost free from the disease. Celiac disease has been reported only rarely in African Americans, but it may be underdiagnosed.

The celiac iceberg
Remarkably, only a small proportion of celiac patients are diagnosed on clinical grounds. Most escape diagnosis unless identified by screening

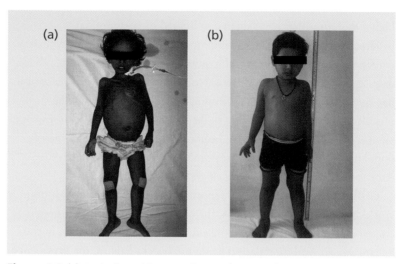

Figure 2.2 (a) An Indian girl presenting at the age of 3.5 years with chronic diarrhea and severe malnutrition. She was positive for celiac autoantibodies, and biopsy from the small intestine showed flat mucosa. (b) An impressive improvement of the nutritional status of this child was evident after 6 months of a gluten-free diet. Reproduced with permission from Catassi C, Yachha S. The global village of celiac disease. In: Fasano A, Troncone R, Branski D, eds. *Frontiers in Celiac Disease. Pediatr Adolesc Med* Basel: Karger, 2008;12:23–31.

with serological markers, such as serum anti-tTG. In developed countries, 5–7 cases remain undiagnosed for each diagnosed case of celiac disease, even though the detection rate is rapidly increasing. These observations have led to the concept of the celiac iceberg, which is made up of:

- a visible part, representing patients who are clinically diagnosed, usually because they are sick
- a far bigger submerged portion that includes all individuals with gluten-sensitive enteropathy who remain undiagnosed, mostly because of atypical complaints or lack of symptoms (Figure 2.4).

The level of the water line, indicative of the ratio of diagnosed to undiagnosed cases, is primarily influenced by the physician's awareness

of the protean manifestations of celiac disease and the threshold for

TABLE 2.1

Prevalence of selected HLA haplotypes predisposing to celiac disease in different populations

Population	Proportion with haplotype (%)	
	DQ2 (*cis*)	DQ8
Saharawi	23.0	2.7
Sardinia	22.4	5.0
Iran	20.0	12.0
Turkey	18.0	22.0
USA	13.1	4.2
Algeria	11.2	2.2
Scandinavia	11.0	15.0
North India	9.0	15.6
Italy	9.0	2.0
Cameroon	9.0	0.6
South African blacks	6.2	2.8
Inuit	6.1	0
Gypsy	6.0	0
Mongolia	5.2	4.4
North American Indians	4.5	25.3
Japan	0.6	7.6
Mexico	0	28.3
Cayapa	0	41.0
Bushman	0	30.2
Highlanders (PNG)	0	0

HLA, human leukocyte antigen; PNG, Papua New Guinea.

requesting serological tests. Current evidence suggests that all celiac patients, regardless of the intensity of their symptoms, are exposed to the long-term complications of this condition, such as anemia, infertility, osteoporosis and lymphoma.

15

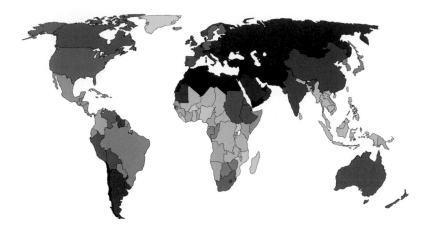

Figure 2.3 Global consumption of wheat per capita per year. The intensity of the color is proportional to consumption. Apart from areas in Sub-Saharan Africa and in the Far East, the consumption of wheat is high worldwide.

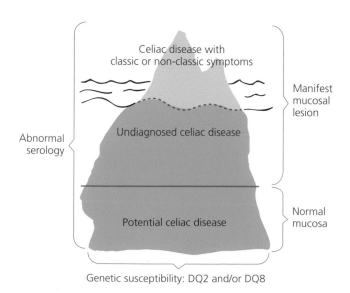

Figure 2.4 The celiac iceberg. For each case of celiac disease diagnosed on clinical grounds there are many others that remain undiscovered (submerged) because of atypical presentation, lack of symptoms or potential stage of the disease.

Risk factors

Genetic. Celiac disease tends to cluster in families (Figure 2.5). In identical twins, the concordance for celiac disease is about 70%, while 5–15% of first-degree relatives are affected. The disease risk for a sibling of an affected individual is about 20-fold higher than for the general population. The familial predisposition depends on human leukocyte antigen (HLA)-related and unrelated genes (see Chapter 3). HLA-DQ2 or HLA-DQ8 genes are necessary for disease development, but are not sufficient in isolation to cause disease. Many other genes involved in adaptive and innate immune responses, intestinal permeability and susceptibility to autoimmune diseases may also influence the risk.

Sex. The prevalence of celiac disease is 1.5–2-fold higher in women, similar to ratios noted for some other autoimmune conditions. It should be noted, however, that these figures are derived from diagnoses made in clinics after biopsy. In general, women are more likely than men to visit their doctor and therefore are likely to have more tests that bring celiac disease to light. When the seroprevalence of celiac disease in the

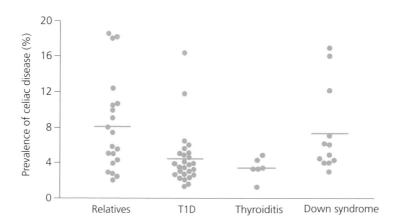

Figure 2.5 The prevalence of celiac disease is increased in different at-risk groups. Each dot in a column indicates the result of a study and a line represents the mean value for that group. T1D, type 1 diabetes.

17

population is considered, this difference between the sexes narrows considerably or disappears.

Diet. The amount and the quality of gluten in the diet may play a role, as well as other dietary components. A protective peptide has been found in durum wheat and beans. Current research is focused on the possible role of early nutritional factors in the later development of celiac disease. The risk of celiac disease seems to be reduced in infants who receive prolonged breastfeeding.

Infections. Intestinal infections can facilitate the immune responses leading to celiac disease. Antibodies directed against the VP7 capsid component of rotaviruses, a common cause of diarrhea worldwide, appear to cross-react with tTG, the major autoantigen in celiac disease.

Other diseases. The prevalence of celiac disease is increased in some patients with other autoimmune disorders, perhaps because of disturbed immunity and shared HLA genotypes (Table 2.2).

Historical perspective

Celiac disease did not exist in the Paleolithic time when hunter–gatherers ate meat, fish, vegetables, pulses and fruit. Cultivation of wheat and barley was first exploited some 10 000 years ago in the so-called 'Fertile Crescent', an area that extends from the Mediterranean Coast on its Western extreme to the great Tigris–Euphrates plain eastward. Farming spread from here and reached the Western edge of Europe some 6000 years ago. According to an old theory, the spread of wheat consumption exerted a negative selective pressure on genes predisposing to celiac disease. This could explain the higher frequency of the disease in Northern Europe, which until relatively recently had a low exposure to cereals. This theory did not survive recent epidemiological developments, as the HLA-related haplotypes predisposing to celiac disease do not show a clear-cut East–West gradient of prevalence. Furthermore, the overall prevalence of celiac disease is not lower in Middle Eastern countries than in Europe, as should be the case if the longer history of agriculture tended to eliminate the genetic predisposing backbone.

TABLE 2.2

Disorders associated with an increased prevalence of celiac disease

Autoimmune disorders

- Type 1 diabetes
- Hashimoto's thyroiditis, Graves' disease
- Sjögren's syndrome
- Hepatitis
- Other (e.g. Addison's disease, vitiligo, immune thrombocytopenic purpura)

Inflammatory bowel disease

- Crohn's disease
- Ulcerative colitis

Genetic disorders

- Down syndrome
- Turner syndrome
- Williams syndrome

Immunoglobulin (Ig)A deficiency

Is the incidence of celiac disease changing?

During the last 2 or 3 decades, the incidence of celiac disease has risen in many countries, generally in association with an increase in the age at diagnosis. This is readily explained by a greater awareness of the many clinical presentations of celiac disease and the availability of accurate screening tests that allow the recognition of atypical or even silent forms of the disease that previously would have been overlooked.

However, it appears that the overall prevalence of celiac disease is also increasing. The prevalence doubled in Finland over 20 years, from 1% in 1978–80 to 2% in 2000–01 (Figure 2.6). According to the hygiene hypothesis, the main factor underlying the increased prevalence of celiac disease and other autoimmune diseases in developed countries

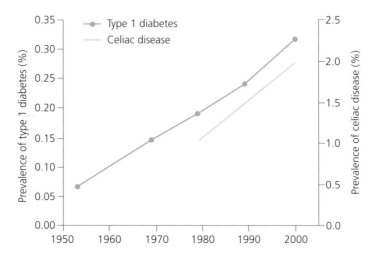

Figure 2.6 Data from Finland illustrate how autoimmune diseases (examples shown are type 1 diabetes and celiac disease) are becoming increasingly prevalent in developed countries. Reproduced from Lohi et al. 2007 with permission from Blackwell Publishing copyright © 2007.

is the reduction in the incidence of infectious diseases. An early childhood infection could down-regulate immunity and suppress autoimmune disorders. Alternatively, the increased prevalence of celiac disease could reflect changes in environmental factors that influence the risk of developing celiac disease, such as the duration of breastfeeding and the amount of gluten ingested.

Is mass screening for celiac disease worthwhile?

Celiac disease would appear to fulfill the criteria for mass screening.

- It is a potentially serious condition that produces significant morbidity.
- Early clinical detection is often difficult.
- If not recognized early, it can present with severe complications, such as malignancy, osteoporosis and neurological problems, which are difficult to manage.
- A gluten-free diet is an effective therapy.
- Sensitive, simple and cheap screening tests are available.

However, the time for mass celiac disease screening has not yet come, as important pieces of information are still lacking. A deeper understanding of the natural history of the condition is needed to ascertain the outcome in the many affected individuals who escape a clinical diagnosis and to determine whether they are susceptible to the complications affecting those patients diagnosed clinically. Given the variable timing of gluten sensitization, the age at which screening should be performed has not been clarified. Furthermore, the negative impact of the gluten-free diet on the long-term psychosocial quality of life should be considered when measuring the cost/benefit of mass screening.

Currently, the best approach to the iceberg of undiagnosed celiac disease is a systematic process of case-finding focused on at risk groups, such as relatives of patients or those with type 1 diabetes, a procedure that minimizes costs and is ethically appropriate. Increased awareness of the clinical polymorphism of celiac disease, coupled with a low threshold for serological testing, can efficiently uncover a large portion of the submerged part of the iceberg. Primary care is the natural setting for selective screening programs.

Key points – epidemiology

- Celiac disease is one of the commonest lifelong disorders in countries populated by people of European origin, affecting around 1% of the general population.
- Celiac disease is increasingly reported from areas of the developing world, especially North Africa, the Middle East and India.
- The prevalence of celiac disease is higher in at-risk groups, such as first-degree relatives, and patients with autoimmune disease or immunoglobulin A deficiency.
- Unless identified by screening with serological markers such as serum anti-tissue transglutaminase antibody, most cases escape diagnosis (and are the submerged part of the celiac iceberg).
- The best approach to identifying undiagnosed cases of celiac disease is a systematic process focused on at-risk groups.

Key references

Catassi C, Kryszak D, Jacques OL et al. Detection of celiac disease in primary care: a multicenter case-finding study in North America. *Am J Gastroenterol* 2007;102:1454–60.

Catassi C, Rätsch IM, Fabiani E et al. Coeliac disease in the year 2000: exploring the iceberg. *Lancet* 1994;343:200–3.

Catassi C, Rätsch IM, Gandolfi L et al. Why is coeliac disease endemic in the people of the Sahara? *Lancet* 1999;354:647–8.

Fasano A, Berti I, Gerarduzzi T et al. Prevalence of celiac disease in at-risk and not-at-risk groups in the United States: a large multicenter study. *Arch Intern Med* 2003;163:286–92.

Lohi S, Mustalahti K, Kaukinen K et al. Increasing prevalence of coeliac disease over time. *Aliment Pharmacol Ther* 2007;26:1217–25.

Mäki M, Mustalahti K, Kokkonen J et al. Prevalence of celiac disease among children in Finland. *N Engl J Med* 2003;348:2517–24.

West J, Logan RF, Hill PG et al. Seroprevalence, correlates, and characteristics of undetected coeliac disease in England. *Gut* 2003;52: 960–5.

Yachha SK. Celiac disease: India on the global map. *J Gastroenterol Hepatol* 2006;21:1511–13.

Celiac disease is a multifactorial disorder that depends on both genetic and environmental factors for expression. The disease appears to be specific to humans, and the lack of an animal model has hampered research. Although the pathogenesis of celiac disease is not yet completely understood, there is evidence to indicate that it is an autoimmune disorder triggered and maintained by an external antigen, namely gluten, in the diet.

Gluten

The term gluten is generically applied to a family of storage proteins found in wheat, rye and barley (8–14% by weight) (Figure 3.1). All the

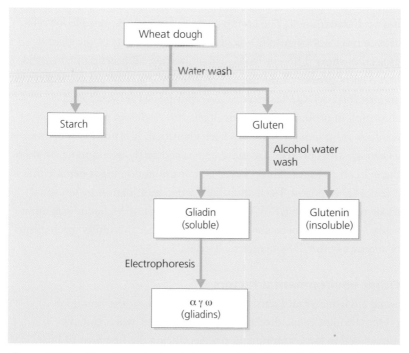

Figure 3.1 Fractionation of wheat showing derivation of gluten and gliadin.

proteins that are harmful to patients with celiac disease are rich in proline and glutamine, and are collectively called prolamins. The prolamin fractions of the various cereals carry different names: gliadin (wheat), secalin (rye) and hordein (barley). The prolamins of oats (avenin) account for only 5–15% of the total seed protein, which could partly explain why celiac patients may tolerate oats in the diet.

The toxic protein fractions of gluten are not only gliadins (alcohol soluble) but also glutenins (alcohol insoluble), with gliadins containing monomeric proteins and glutenins containing aggregated proteins. The protein components and amino acid sequences of gliadins and glutenins are similar and repetitive. In a single wheat variety, there are approximately 45 different gliadins, which can be subdivided into α, γ, and ω subfractions according to their electrophoretic mobility. This complexity has made gluten a difficult substance to investigate within the context of celiac disease.

The sequence of A-gliadin, a protein made up of 266 amino acids, has been determined. The amino acid sequence(s) responsible for celiac disease have not been fully elucidated. Different parts of the gliadin molecules show different biological properties, all potentially involved in the pathogenesis of the disease (Figure 3.2). Several human leukocyte antigen (HLA)-DQ2-restricted T-cell epitopes have been found clustering in proline-rich regions of gliadin. A gliadin peptide of 33 residues, α2-gliadin 57–89, has been identified. It is produced by normal gastrointestinal proteolysis and contains six partly overlapping copies of three T-cell epitopes. This 33-mer is an immunodominant peptide that is a remarkably potent T-cell stimulator after deamidation by intestinal tissue transglutaminase (tTG). Other sequences of A-gliadin (e.g. amino acids 31–43) have been shown to activate innate immunity mechanisms or interact with CD8+ cytotoxic T cells.

Other environmental factors

Some environmental factors may affect the risk or the timing of presentation of celiac disease. The risk is greater when gluten is introduced in large amounts in the diet during the first year of life. Conversely, breastfeeding has a consistently protective effect; in particular, the risk of celiac disease is reduced if children are still

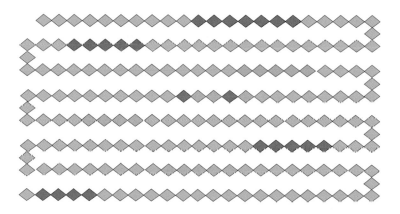

Figure 3.2 A gliadin protein shown as a simple chain of amino acids. The regions that act as immunogenic epitopes are shown in red shades, with the relative antigenicity shown by intensity of color. A protective peptide that can reduce the gluten-induced damage, recently identified in durum wheat, is shown in blue.

breastfed when dietary gluten is introduced. It is unclear if breastfeeding prevents celiac disease or merely delays onset.

Recent studies have shown that in children prone to celiac disease as a result of having HLA-DQ2 or -DQ8 genes, initial exposure to wheat, barley and rye in the first 3 months of life significantly increases the risk of the development of autoantibodies associated with celiac disease compared with exposure at a later age. Although the risk associated with later introduction of gluten (older than 7 months) is disputed, prospective studies being carried out in newborn infants who are first-degree relatives of patients with celiac disease should clarify this issue.

The autoimmune mechanism leading to celiac enteropathy could be triggered by intestinal infection. In this regard, an antibody directed against a rotavirus capsid protein (VP7) has been found in patients with active celiac disease. This antibody recognizes self-antigens (tTG) and can increase intestinal permeability and induce monocyte activation.

Cigarette smoking appears to protect against the development of celiac disease.

Genetics

Celiac disease is a multifactorial condition with unparalleled evidence of the pivotal role of *HLA-DQA1*05-DQB1*02* (DQ2) and *DQA1*03-DQB1*0302* (DQ8) genes in disease predisposition. HLA-DQ is a family of genes encoding heterodimer-forming proteins that have a role in antigen recognition by the antigen-presenting cells. The *HLA-DQA1* gene encodes the α subunit of the αβ-heterodimer and the *HLA-DQB1* gene encodes the β subunit (Figure 3.3). Celiac disease is strongly associated with the HLA variant DQ2.5 *(DQA1*05/DQB1*02)*. The monomer subunits of the HLA-DQ heterodimer can be encoded on the same chromosome (*cis*) or on separate chromosomes (*trans*) (Figure 3.4). Individuals with a double copy of DQ2 *(DQB1*02)* have increased susceptibility to celiac disease (Figure 3.5).

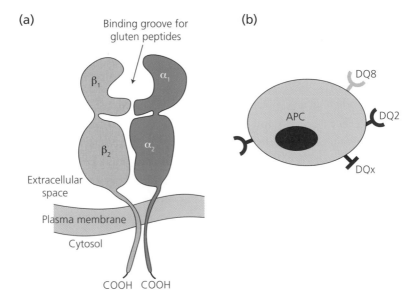

(a)

Binding groove for gluten peptides

β₁ α₁

β₂ α₂

Extracellular space

Plasma membrane

Cytosol

COOH   COOH

(b)

DQ8

APC

DQ2

DQx

Figure 3.3 Human leukocyte antigen (HLA)-DQ genes encode heterodimer-forming proteins. (a) The heterodimer has a role in antigen recognition by the antigen-presenting cell (APC). (b) APCs from individuals lacking the DQ2 and/or DQ8 receptors (DQx) are unable to link the activated gluten peptides and celiac disease is not triggered.

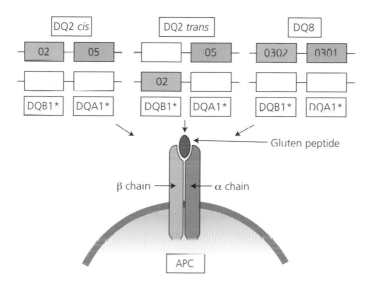

Figure 3.4 The DQ2 (in *cis* and *trans* configuration) and the DQ8 haplotypes.

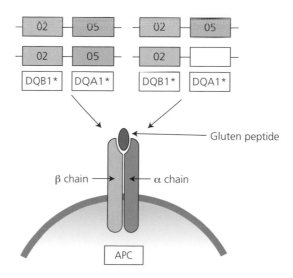

Figure 3.5 A double copy of DQ2 (*DQB1*02*) increases susceptibility to celiac disease. It has also been associated with an increased risk of refractory celiac disease.

27

This genotype has also been associated with an increased risk of refractory celiac disease. The most likely mechanism to explain the association with HLA class II genes is that the DQ heterodimers bind to gliadin peptide fragments and present these to T cells. The requirements for peptide binding to the HLA molecules have outlined the importance of proline spacing and gluten deamidation in this process.

HLA alone does not explain overall genetic susceptibility because the concordance rate between identical twins (approximately 70%) is higher than that between HLA-identical siblings (30%). It is likely that additional genetic factors influence disease propensity. There is an association with the tumor necrosis factor (TNF)-2 allele, this polymorphism being associated with increased TNFα expression. Involvement of the gene for the negative costimulatory molecule cytotoxic T-lymphocyte-associated protein 4 (CTLA4) or a neighboring gene has been highlighted.

A series of whole-genome screening studies have been performed in patients with celiac disease. A provisional list of loci predisposing to celiac disease includes *CELIAC1* (also known as *HLA-DQB1*) on chromosome 6 (HLA-DQ2 and HLA-DQ8), *CELIAC2* on chromosome 5q31-33, *CELIAC3* on chromosome 2q33 (containing the T lymphocyte regulatory gene *CTLA4*) and *CELIAC4* (or *MYO9B*), the myosin IXB gene on chromosome 19p13.1. *MYO9B* encodes an unconventional myosin molecule that may have a role in actin remodeling in epithelial enterocytes. It has been hypothesized that this genetic variant might lead to an impaired intestinal barrier, which could allow the passage of immunogenic gluten peptides. Although the non-HLA genes together contribute more to genetic susceptibility than do the HLA genes, the contribution from each single predisposing non-HLA gene appears to be modest.

Intestinal barrier

Under physiological circumstances, intestinal epithelia are almost impermeable to macromolecules such as gliadin. In celiac disease, paracellular permeability is enhanced and the integrity of the tight junction (TJ) system is compromised. The upregulation of zonulin – a recently described intestinal peptide involved in TJ regulation – appears to be responsible, at least in part, for the characteristic of increased gut permeability in celiac disease. Following engagement of the chemokine receptor CXCR3, specific A-gliadin peptides cause zonulin release. This is followed by a protein kinase C-mediated polymerization of intracellular actin filaments, which are directly connected to TJ complex proteins, thereby regulating epithelial permeability. Further, persistent presence of inflammatory mediators such as TNFα and interferon (IFN)γ has been shown to increase the permeability across the endothelial and epithelial layers. This suggests that the initial breach of the intestinal barrier function caused by zonulin can be perpetuated by the inflammatory process after gliadin has reached the submucosa. Gliadin activates zonulin signaling, resulting in immediate reduction of intestinal barrier function and passage of gliadin into the subepithelial compartment. This process depends on the presence of the zonulin receptor, but is independent of individual genetic predisposition, suggesting that gliadin-induced zonulin-mediated paracellular permeability could be required but is not sufficient to develop the autoimmune process typical of celiac disease.

Jejunal mucosa

Abnormalities of the jejunal mucosa are the hallmark of celiac disease. The diagnosis is based on characteristic appearances of the enterocytes, villi, crypts and the inflammatory cell infiltrate in the mucosa.

Normal mucosa. Digitate villi, leaf forms and ridges are seen in normal jejunal mucosa (Figures 3.6a and 3.7a). When viewed by transmission light microscopy, the villi constitute 65–80% of the total mucosal thickness, while the crypts make up the remainder (Figure 3.8). The villi are covered by a single layer of columnar cells called enterocytes, which have a basally situated nucleus and a well-marked brush border. Cells migrate up the crypts to replace enterocytes, which are being continually lost from the villus tips into the bowel lumen. In the epithelium, the sparse cellular infiltrate is made up almost exclusively of intraepithelial lymphocytes; in the lamina propria, it is composed mainly of plasma cells, lymphocytes and macrophages.

(a)

(b)

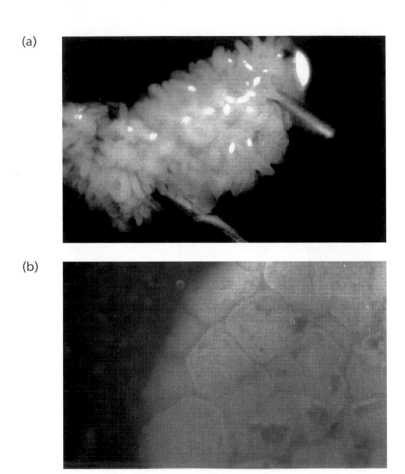

Figure 3.6 (a) Normal jejunal mucosa showing finger-like villi. (b) The flat mucosa of celiac disease showing the characteristic mosaic appearance.

Typical celiac mucosa appears flat with a mosaic pattern under the light-dissecting microscope (Figure 3.6b). Histologically, there are no structures in the mucosa that can be identified as villi (Figure 3.9). The crypts are hypertrophied and open directly on to the mucosal surface.

The cells constituting the mucosal surface are cuboidal and appear stratified, and the brush border is poorly developed. A dense infiltrate of lymphocytes and plasma cells is found in the lamina propria and the intraepithelial lymphocytes are increased in number. The openings of the

(a)

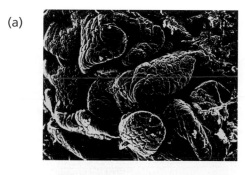

Figure 3.7 (a) Normal jejunal mucosa with leaf-shaped villi protruding into the intestinal lumen (× 100). (b) The typical flat mucosa and crater-shaped openings of the crypts in untreated celiac disease (× 150). Reproduced courtesy of S Cinti and M Morroni, Morphology Institute of Università Politecnica delle Marche, Ancona, Italy.

(b)

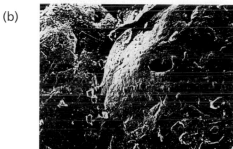

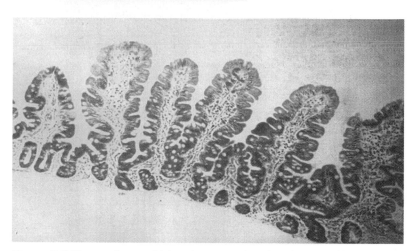

Figure 3.8 Biopsy of normal jejunal mucosa showing digitate villi.

crypts directly on to the surface of the mucosa are shown particularly well by scanning electron microscopy (Figure 3.7b). Although a number of other conditions may cause a flat biopsy, such findings in an adult living in the Western world are almost certain to indicate celiac disease.

31

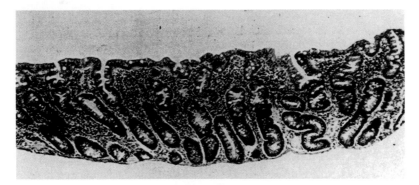

Figure 3.9 Jejunal biopsy from a patient with untreated celiac disease. Villi are absent and the crypts hypertrophied. Intraepithelial lymphocytes are increased in number and a heavy infiltrate of plasma cells and lymphocytes is evident in the lamina propria.

Spectrum of gluten sensitivity and mucosal pathology

It is clear from observations made in patients with dermatitis herpetiformis and in relatives of patients with celiac disease, as well as from gluten-challenge studies, that the classic appearances of celiac disease form only one facet of gluten sensitivity and that less severe lesions can occur. The typical flat mucosa found in active celiac disease is likely to be the end-stage lesion of T-cell-dependent immune reactivity that progresses through several phases of mucosal pathology from type 1 to type 3, as outlined in Chapter 1 (see Table 1.1 and Figure 1.1).

There is a dynamic relationship between the pathology types with progression in either direction. An important factor influencing the severity of the enteropathy is the amount of gluten ingested, but other factors include gastrointestinal infections and the stresses of surgery or pregnancy. The mucosal pathology of gluten sensitivity and celiac disease is even wider than this, as some patients with dermatitis herpetiformis have biopsies that appear indistinguishable from normal (Type 0), while in others an irreversible atrophic lesion associated with jejunoileitis and enteropathy-associated T-cell lymphoma can occur.

Extent of disease. Although celiac enteropathy is typically confined to the duodenum and proximal jejunum, the length of the damaged intestine can vary. The residual unaffected bowel could undergo functional

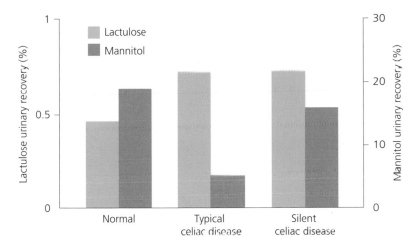

Figure 3.10 Results of the lactulose/mannitol intestinal permeability test suggest a possible explanation for the different expressions of celiac disease. Lactulose urinary recovery (which may reflect paracellular permeability) is increased in both typical and silent forms of the disease because of the enteropathy. However, mannitol recovery (which is directly related to the absorptive surface area) is reduced only in typical forms. This indicates that the mucosal damage extends for a shorter distance down the bowel in clinically silent cases. (For more information on the intestinal permeability test see page 66.)

hypertrophy and thus determine the balance between clinical 'silence' and symptoms. This possibility has been confirmed by a dual-sugar intestinal permeability study. Children with typical celiac disease usually show a decrease in mannitol urinary recovery, which is thought to reflect the decrease in the overall intestinal mucosa surface. Individuals with silent celiac disease, however, have a mannitol urinary recovery result within normal limits (Figure 3.10), which suggests that they remain symptom-free because the damaged area of intestinal mucosa is small.

Adaptive and innate immunologic response to gluten

Celiac enteropathy is most likely the result of immune-mediated damage to the small-intestinal mucosa. Both adaptive and innate immune responses are involved, driven by different gliadin peptides (Figure 3.11). 33

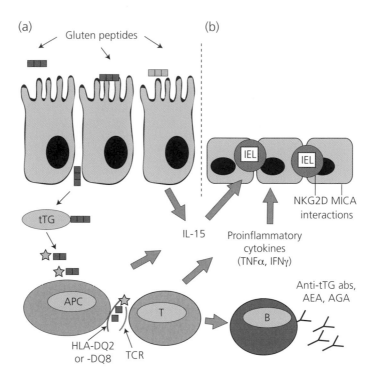

Figure 3.11 (a) The adaptive and innate immune response in the small-intestinal mucosa leading to (b) celiac enteropathy. Some gluten peptides, e.g. fragment 57–89 of α2-gliadin (red), cross the intestinal barrier at the paracellular level where they are modified by tissue transglutaminase (tTG). Deamidated gluten peptides (with stars) interact with HLA-DQ2 or -DQ8 receptors located on the intestinal antigen-presenting cells (APC), activating an adaptive T-cell response via the T-cell receptor (TCR), with proinflammatory cytokine production and a B-lymphocyte response leading to autoantibody synthesis. Other gluten peptides, e.g. fragment 31–43 (brown), stimulate an innate response by upregulating the synthesis of interleukin (IL)-15 by epithelial cells and lamina propria mononuclear cells. IL-15 has a direct action on intraepithelial lymphocytes (IELs) that promotes their survival and accumulation. Cytotoxicity of the enterocytes occurs by the release of proinflammatory cytokines, particularly interferon-γ (IFNγ) by antigen-specific T cells and directly by IELs via NKG2D (on IELs) and MICA (on enterocytes), both of which are upregulated by IL-15. AEA, anti-endomysial antibody; AGA, anti-gliadin antibody; TCR, T-cell receptor; TNF, tumor necrosis factor.

The structural and immunohistological features of the celiac enteropathy closely resemble those seen in animal models of T-cell mucosal injury, such as allograft rejection, graft-versus-host disease or experimental giardiasis.

A ubiquitous enzyme, tTG, is the major autoantigen responsible for anti-endomysial antibody positivity. Gliadin is an excellent substrate for intestinal tTG because of its high glutamine content (about 40%). In the lamina propria, tTG converts glutamine in gliadin peptides into negatively charged glutamic acid, a process called deamidation. After deamidation, the affinity of gluten peptides for HLA receptors located on the membrane of antigen-presenting cells is greatly increased. The interaction between gliadin peptides and HLA receptors activates an adaptive immune response mediated by intestinal T cells.

The pattern of cytokines produced by lymphocytes after gliadin activation is dominated by IFNγ; however, interleukin (IL)-10 is also upregulated. On the other hand, the gliadin-derived fragment p31–43 induces an innate response mediated by IL-15, which is secreted by enterocytes and activated dendritic cells in the lamina propria. IL-15 could be the main factor orchestrating the selective expansion of intraepithelial lymphocytes, particularly T-cell receptor (TCR)γδ and CD8 TCRα/β lymphocytes bearing the CD94 natural killer (NK) receptor. Recent studies pinpoint the fundamental role of the innate immune response in damaging the intestinal mucosa in celiac disease, primarily by causing intraepithelial lymphocyte-mediated cytolysis of the epithelium.

The pathogenesis of autoimmune disease

Increased intestinal permeability is likely to be a factor in the pathogenesis of a variety of autoimmune diseases. A common denominator of these diseases is the presence of several pre-existing circumstances that lead to an autoimmune process. The first is a genetic susceptibility for the host immune system to recognize, and potentially misinterpret, an environmental antigen presented to the body (e.g. within the gastrointestinal tract). Second, the host must be exposed to the antigen. Finally, the antigen must be presented to the mucosal immune system following its paracellular passage from the lumen to the submucosa, normally prevented by TJ competency. In many cases, increased intestinal permeability precedes disease and causes an abnormality in antigen delivery that triggers the multi-organ process that leads to the autoimmune response. Based on these findings, it is possible to formulate a hypothesis to explain the pathogenesis of autoimmune diseases that encompasses the following three key points.

- Autoimmune diseases involve a miscommunication between innate and adaptive immunity.
- Molecular mimicry or bystander effects are probably not involved in the pathogenesis of autoimmune diseases. Rather, the continuous stimulus of non-self antigens (environmental triggers) is likely to be necessary to perpetuate the process. This concept implies that the autoimmune response can, theoretically, be stopped and/or reversed if the interplay between autoimmune predisposing genes and trigger(s) can be prevented or eliminated.
- In addition to genetic predisposition and exposure to the triggering non-self antigen, the protective function of mucosal barriers that interface with the environment (mainly gastrointestinal and lung mucosa) is lost.

Current evidence suggests that any autoimmune disease, including celiac disease, needs four classes of genes, i.e. genes involved in:

- antigen presentation, namely some HLA class II haplotypes (e.g. DQ2)
- innate and/or adaptive immunity other than HLA: these are the genes that dictate the host response to intestinal microorganisms, supporting the notion that the role of the microbiome in the pathogenesis of autoimmune diseases is limited to that of 'instigator' rather than trigger. This is the reason why attempts to identify a specific microorganism as a cause of autoimmunity have so far failed
- inflammation
- intestinal barrier control.

There is little variability in the first group, as HLA class II genes are almost always involved. There is much more variability in the other three classes of genes. This explains the heterogeneous nature and, therefore, the low weight (meaning the necessity to be there) of these additional genes when considered singularly. However, if considered as a category, their weight increases dramatically. Therefore, it is likely that the search for 'the gene(s)' of autoimmunity will remain elusive, as even in the same disease (i.e. celiac disease) it is entirely possible that it is not always the same gene that dictates intestinal permeability or immune modulation.

Celiac disease represents the best model to support this scheme. The upregulation of the zonulin innate pathway induced by exposure to the antigenic trigger, gluten, causes increased intestinal permeability leading to the passage of gluten through to the submucosa. There, an inflammatory environment is initiated by the interaction of submucosal macrophages with gluten, leading to activation of the adaptive immune response with the subsequent secretion of cytokines and the production of autoantibodies (with specificity for tTG). Ultimately, intestinal mucosal damage occurs. Once gluten is removed from the diet, serum zonulin levels decrease, intestinal permeability normalizes, autoantibody titers return to the normal range, the autoimmune process shuts off and the intestinal damage that represents the biological outcome of the autoimmune process completely heals.

Key points – pathophysiology

- Gluten contains several toxic epitopes that can activate innate immunity, adaptive immunity or intestinal barrier dysfunction in celiac disease.
- Celiac disease is a unique autoimmune disease because both the major genetic factors (HLA-DQ2 and -DQ8) and etiologic agent (dietary gluten) for susceptibility are known.
- While the environmental factor is clearly identified, the genetic makeup remains extremely complex and variable from one population to another; the exception is the HLA class II genes, which are common to all patients with celiac disease.
- Besides the genetic makeup and the exposure to gluten, loss of intestinal barrier function seems to be a third element involved in the pathogenesis of celiac disease.
- As a result of the aberrant immune response to gliadin, several cytokines activating both T helper cell (Th)1 and Th17 responses are evoked.
- The outcome of the autoimmune process is damage to the mucosa of the upper small intestine that reverses when gluten is removed from the diet.

Key references

Benahmed M, Meresse B, Arnulf B et al. Inhibition of TGF-beta signaling by IL-15: a new role for IL-15 in the loss of immune homeostasis in celiac disease. *Gastroenterology* 2007;132:994–1008.

Branski D, Fasano A, Troncone R. Latest developments in the pathogenesis and treatment of celiac disease. *J Pediatr* 2006;149:295–300.

Harris KM, Fasano A, Mann DL. Cutting edge: IL-1 controls the IL-23 response induced by gliadin, the etiologic agent in celiac disease. *J Immunol* 2008;181:4457–60.

Jabri B, Sollid LM. Mechanisms of disease: immunopathogenesis of celiac disease. *Nat Clin Pract Gastroenterol Hepatol* 2006;3: 516–25.

Koning F. Celiac disease: caught between a rock and a hard place. *Gastroenterology* 2005;129: 1294–301.

Lammers KM, Lu R, Brownley J et al. Gliadin induces an increase in intestinal permeability and zonulin release by binding to the chemokine receptor CXCR3. *Gastroenterology* 2008;135:194–204.

Stepniak D, Koning F. Celiac disease – sandwiched between innate and adaptive immunity. *Hum Immunol* 2006;67:460–8.

Wolters VM, Wijmenga C. Genetic background of celiac disease and its clinical implications. *Am J Gastroenterol* 2008;103:190–5.

Clinical manifestations

Celiac disease presents with a wide spectrum of clinical manifestations in children and adults. The diagnosis will often be overlooked unless it is actively considered when it is a possibility in patients with unexplained clinical and laboratory features (Table 4.1).

Factors affecting clinical presentation

The reasons why the clinical expression of celiac disease is so highly variable and why presentation can occur at any time in life, from

---

TABLE 4.1

Features suggestive of celiac disease

- History of celiac disease in childhood or in the family
- Recurrent abdominal pain in childhood
- Delayed puberty
- Short stature
- History of rickets
- Non-specific ill health
- Weight loss
- Diarrhea
- Recurrent mouth ulcers
- Chronic fatigue
- Autoimmune diseases
- Anemia, raised mean corpuscular volume, folate and iron deficiency

- Hypocalcemia
- Osteoporosis and osteomalacia
- Infertility and recurrent miscarriages
- IgA deficiency
- Splenic atrophy and hyposplenism
- Bleeding tendency
- Unexplained neurological disturbances
- Malabsorption syndrome
- Unexplained hypertransaminasemia
- Down, Turner or Williams syndromes
- Alopecia areata

IgA, immunoglobulin A.

infancy to very old age, are not fully understood. A number of factors have, however, been implicated.

Age. The symptoms of malabsorption are usually more marked during the first years of life and then gradually decrease. This is probably a reflection of the decreasing ratio between the length of the diseased proximal and the unaffected distal small intestine.

Amount of gluten ingested. The probability that a patient will have a severe enteropathy, and therefore the clinical manifestations of celiac disease, increases with the amount of gluten that is eaten.

Genetic influences. Particular combinations of HLA and non-HLA genes may predispose to earlier disease onset and more severe clinical manifestations. HLA-DQ2 homozygosity in patients with celiac disease is associated with an increased risk of developing intestinal lymphoma (see Chapter 3).

Intestinal infections. The absorptive defect caused by celiac disease in the proximal small intestine can be masked by compensation in the distal ileum. The diffuse impairment of intestinal function caused by an intestinal infection can precipitate the onset of diarrhea and unmask celiac disease.

Pregnancy. Occasionally, celiac disease becomes clinically manifest during pregnancy or soon after childbirth.

Surgery. The stress of an operation (e.g. partial gastrectomy or hysterectomy) can precipitate symptoms of celiac disease.

Lymphoma. The development of intestinal lymphoma may unmask celiac disease.

Presentation in children and adolescents

Typical celiac disease. The typical child with celiac disease presents between 6 and 24 months of age with impaired growth, abnormal stools, abdominal distension, muscle wasting and hypotonia, poor appetite and unhappy behavior (Figure 4.1); pallor and edema may also be seen. The onset of symptoms is gradual and usually characterized by a time lag of some months after weaning. Velocity of weight gain slowly decreases and weight loss then follows (Figure 4.2). The stools

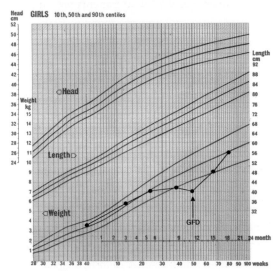

Figure 4.1 A child aged 15 months with typical celiac disease. He is severely malnourished with abdominal distension and edema.

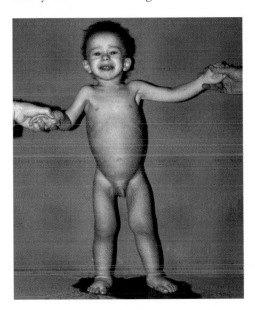

Figure 4.2 The 'parabolic' weight curve of a child with typical celiac disease. The child gained weight following the introduction of a gluten-free diet (GFD).

41

become frequent, pale, soft, bulky and offensive. Occasionally, constipation is a prominent feature. Vomiting commonly occurs in very young infants. Manifestations of vitamin D deficiency, such as rickets and hypocalcemia, or the so-called 'celiac crisis', an emergency situation with watery diarrhea, dehydration and shock, have become rare in developed countries.

In many European countries, typical cases of celiac disease represent 20–30% of new pediatric diagnoses but are less frequent in North America. The reason for this difference is not clear, but could be related to lower gluten intake in American infants. When diagnostic facilities are not readily available (e.g. in some developing countries), long-standing untreated celiac disease is characterized by stunting, pubertal delay, chronic diarrhea, abdominal distension and severe iron-deficiency anemia.

Atypical celiac disease is usually seen in older children and features of overt malabsorption are absent. The symptoms and signs may be intestinal or extraintestinal.

Intestinal features may include recurrent abdominal pain, irritable-bowel-like symptoms (e.g. recurrent diarrhea), dental enamel defects (Figure 4.3), and recurrent aphthous stomatitis.

Extraintestinal features. Between 6 and 12% of patients with iron-deficiency anemia attending a hematology clinic are found to have celiac disease; this anemia is typically resistant to oral iron therapy. Isolated increase of serum aminotransferase level, caused by mild non-progressive liver inflammation, is a common presentation of active celiac disease.

Short stature and delayed puberty can be the primary manifestation in an otherwise healthy child. Celiac disease is the most common organic cause of slow height gain and is far more common than growth hormone (GH) deficiency. The endocrinologic pattern usually includes delayed bone age, either normal or blunted GH response to stimulatory tests and low levels of insulin-like growth factor-1. Treatment with a gluten-free diet (GFD) often leads to complete catch-up growth within 2–3 years. If no catch-up growth occurs after 12 months of starting a GFD, an associated and transient GH deficiency should be suspected. In

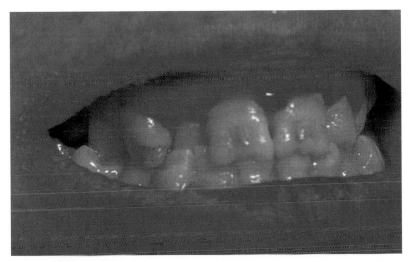

Figure 4.3 Dental enamel defects in a patient with newly diagnosed celiac disease. Reproduced courtesy of A Ventura, Department of Paediatrics, University of Trieste, Italy.

these patients, a period of GH replacement therapy as well as a GFD may improve the final height.

Joint disease. Celiac disease can also present with joint disease. This takes the form of pain and stiffness affecting mainly the shoulders, elbows, knees and hands.

Silent celiac disease has been recognized increasingly since the introduction of serological tests to screen or find cases within groups. This often occurs in individuals with a family history of celiac disease, or in those with associated autoimmune disorders (e.g. type 1 diabetes) or genetic conditions (e.g. Down, Turner or Williams syndromes). A thorough history and investigation will, however, reveal a low-grade illness in many of these individuals.

Common features are:
- behavioral disturbances, such as irritability and impaired school performance
- impaired physical fitness and chronic fatigue
- iron deficiency with or without anemia
- reduced bone mineral density (Figure 4.4).

(a)

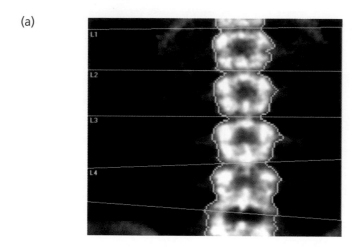

(b)

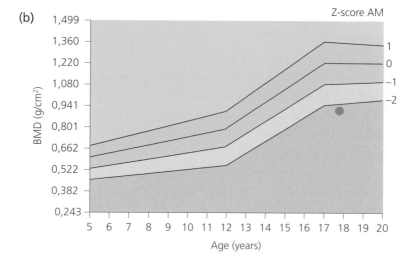

Figure 4.4 Dual X-ray absorptiometry of the spine of a 17-year-old boy
with active celiac disease shows (a) the image of the lumbar vertebrae
and (b) the plot of bone mineral density (BMD) measurement against
a reference curve. The value (pink dot) lies 2 standard deviations
(SD) below the average, and should be considered low for chronological
age. Reproduced courtesy of S Mora, San Raffaele Scientific Institute, Milan,
Italy.

Presentation in adults

Patients with overt malabsorption and severe symptoms of celiac disease are still seen, but most now present with trivial or non-specific complaints. The diagnosis is often only suspected from abnormalities found on routine blood tests, particularly anemia, a raised mean corpuscular volume (MCV), iron and folate deficiency and hypocalcemia, which, together with hypophosphatemia and elevated alkaline phosphatase, indicates osteomalacia. Some cases are identified from family studies or screening programs.

While many patients consider themselves to have mild or even no symptoms, they are often only able to recognize the full extent of their ill health retrospectively, following the benefits conferred by a GFD. Many will find that they had accepted a significant degree of illness as normal. Thus, as in pediatric practice, adults may present with typical or atypical symptoms or with silent celiac disease.

Clinical features. The features of celiac disease at presentation are protean (Table 4.2 and Figure 4.5). Diarrhea is the most common symptom, but only affects just over 50% of patients, is of variable duration (40% of patients < 1 year and 35% < 5 years) and can present acutely in a previously well person. Lethargy and tiredness, with or without anemia or other features, and weight loss are also common symptoms. Abdominal distension affects about one-third of patients. Altered bowel habit and bloating may be mistakenly attributed to irritable bowel syndrome.

Elevated levels of serum aminotransferases are common in untreated celiac disease, affecting about half of all adults with celiac disease, and are corrected after 6–12 months of a strict GFD.

Conversely, celiac disease occurs in about 10% of those with unexplained hypertransaminasemia. This abnormality is an expression of a mild liver dysfunction with a histological picture of non-specific reactive hepatitis (celiac hepatitis). Rarely, a more severe liver injury, characterized by a cryptogenic chronic hepatitis or liver cirrhosis, is present. In these patients, liver damage can still improve with a GFD.

Peripheral neuropathy, ataxia indicating spinocerebellar degeneration, arthropathy, infertility and bleeding disorders are less

TABLE 4.2

Presenting features of celiac disease

General

- Short stature
- Weight loss
- Lassitude/lethargy
- Edema
- Clubbing
- Koilonychia
- Bruising

Gastrointestinal

- Anorexia, nausea, vomiting
- Glossitis, mouth ulcers
- Abdominal distension and pain
- Flatulence and flatus
- Diarrhea, constipation

Psychiatric

- Depression
- Anxiety

Neurological

- Peripheral neuropathy
- Ataxia
- Epilepsy

Hematologic

- Anemia
- Folic acid and iron deficiency
- Raised mean corpuscular volume
- Hemorrhagic manifestations

Biochemical

- Reduced serum calcium, raised alkaline phosphatase
- Increased serum aminotransferase levels

Reproduction

- Infertility
- Recurrent miscarriages

Musculoskeletal

- Osteomalacia, osteoporosis, bone pain
- Myopathy
- Cramps, tetany, paresthesia

Renal

- Nocturnal diuresis

Skin

- Dermatitis herpetiformis
- Pigmentation

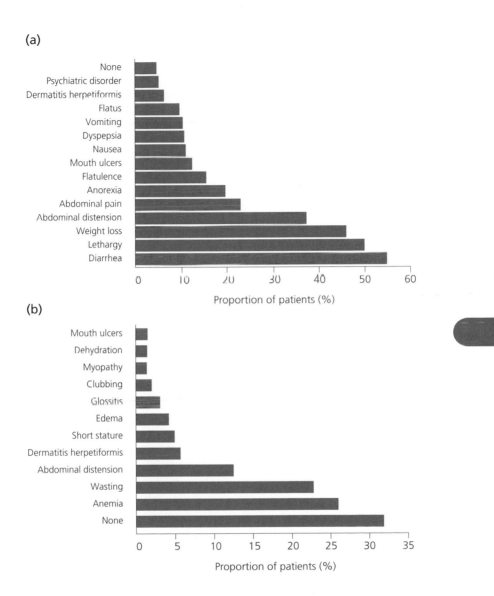

Figure 4.5 (a) Symptoms and (b) signs at presentation in 352 adult patients with celiac disease diagnosed in one clinic.

common presentations. In about 4% of cases, celiac disease presents during pregnancy or within weeks or months of giving birth. It is noteworthy that only about 5% of patients are asymptomatic if a

47

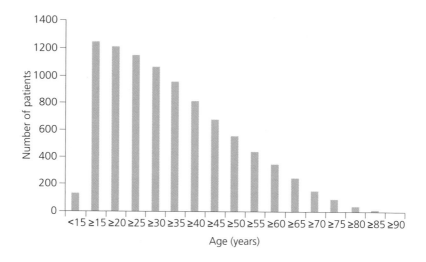

Figure 4.6 Age distribution of patients with celiac disease at diagnosis attending the Derby Adult Coeliac Clinic, UK.

careful history is elicited; there are no abnormal signs in about one-third of patients.

The elderly. Celiac disease is being increasingly diagnosed in later life and, today, about 25% of cases are diagnosed in patients over 60 years of age and 10% in those aged over 70 years (Figure 4.6). Contrary to common belief, 95% of these patients manage a GFD well and enjoy a much improved quality of life.

Associated autoimmune disorders

Many disorders occur in association with celiac disease. These can cause diagnostic difficulties if, rather than prompting a search for a second diagnosis, the clinical features are attributed to the established diagnosis.

Disturbed immunity in celiac disease may predispose affected individuals to other disorders that also have an immunologic etiology. HLA patterns common to celiac and other autoimmune diseases (e.g. HLA-DQ8 and -DQ2) are also likely to be of importance. Increased intestinal permeability, a feature of untreated celiac disease, may allow antigens, including microbial agents, access to the immune system and may be important in provoking liver disease. The prevalence of the conditions coexisting with celiac disease is difficult to determine because studies are often carried out in referral centers or patients are from selected groups, and this introduces bias. In addition, many patients with celiac disease are undiagnosed in the community and if it were possible to consider these, the prevalence figures might be greatly diluted. Recent studies do not confirm the possibility that the prevalence of autoimmune disorders is related to the duration of exposure to gluten. The disorders most commonly associated with celiac disease are shown in Table 4.3.

Type 1 diabetes mellitus is the commonest and best-researched association. The diagnosis of celiac disease may precede that of diabetes, but in 90% of cases diabetes is diagnosed first. Screening studies have revealed that the prevalence of celiac disease among children with diabetes is about 4.5% and in adults around 3.5%.

At the time of screening most children do not have gastrointestinal symptoms, but failure to thrive, malabsorption, growth failure, unstable diabetes, unexplained anemia and elevated aminotransferase activity indicate that celiac disease may be present. Adults may have symptoms of untreated celiac disease such as lethargy, bloating, vomiting and diarrhea as well as recurrent hypoglycemia, anemia, and folate and iron deficiency. The proportions of children and adults with symptoms and signs differ widely in the many reports available, and this probably reflects how carefully the signs and symptoms were looked for. It is

---

TABLE 4.3

The most common immunologic disorders associated with celiac disease

- Type 1 diabetes mellitus
- Autoimmune liver diseases
- Thyroid disorders
- Ulcerative colitis
- Crohn's disease
- Sjögren's syndrome
- IgA deficiency

IgA, immunoglobulin A.

likely that some patients were regarded as asymptomatic when they were not.

A careful history will often reveal subtle complaints consistent with celiac disease. Furthermore, ill health may only be recognized retrospectively, following the benefits conferred by a GFD. Probably about 50% of patients have symptoms. It should not be forgotten that those with celiac disease may subsequently develop type 1 diabetes.

As celiac disease commonly occurs in type 1 diabetes, a case for offering screening to all patients with type 1 diabetes can be made. Those who have suggestive symptoms are likely to accept and if the diagnosis is confirmed they should be referred to a sympathetic dietician who is skilled in managing diabetes and a GFD. Those who regard themselves as asymptomatic may be reluctant to be screened, but the issues should be fully discussed so that they can make an informed choice.

A single negative screening test for celiac disease does not rule out the disease for life, so serial testing is required. A possible program would entail screening at the diagnosis of diabetes, then yearly for 3 years, then at 5 years and 5-yearly thereafter, or at any time if there are clinical indications. Demonstration of the absence of HLA-DQ2 and HLA-DQ8 would eliminate the diagnosis of celiac disease.

A GFD improves symptoms related to celiac disease. Many experience improved wellbeing and vitality, even some who regarded themselves as asymptomatic before the diet was commenced. Growth rate may increase in children. The effect of a GFD on control of diabetes varies from no effect to improved control with fewer hypoglycemic episodes. Many patients detected by screening may be completely asymptomatic and tend to abandon the diet, which they regard as another imposition on an already difficult lifestyle.

Type 2 diabetes occurs in celiac disease, but with a frequency much as that expected in the general population.

Thyroid disease. Celiac disease is associated with hypothyroidism, thyroiditis and hyperthyroidism. Up to 12% of patients with celiac disease may have overt hypothyroidism and 7% hyperthyroidism.

12% of patients with celiac disease have Hashimoto's thyroiditis and 5% with Hashimoto's thyroiditis have celiac disease. It is important to be aware of these associations because those with celiac disease may mistakenly have their symptoms of, for example, weight loss, lethargy and diarrhea attributed to a relapse of celiac disease ascribed to dietary indiscretions rather than to the presence of thyroid disease. In children, Hashimoto's thyroiditis is more common in school-age girls and may also be found not uncommonly in children who are already following a GFD. As clinical manifestations of thyroiditis in children are often mild or absent, serological screening with anti-thyroperoxidase and anti-thyroglobulin antibodies is indicated in the follow-up of girls with treated celiac disease.

Autoimmune liver disease. Celiac disease is present in 3–7% of those with primary biliary cirrhosis, autoimmune hepatitis and primary sclerosing cholangitis. A GFD does not appear to influence the course of these diseases.

Pulmonary diseases. Diffuse lung disease occurs in celiac disease. Fibrosing alveolitis, bird fancier's lung and farmer's lung are found, but the significance of these associations is not clear. There may be a link between celiac disease and idiopathic pulmonary hemosiderosis.

Heart diseases. An association between celiac disease and autoimmune myocarditis or idiopathic dilated cardiomyopathy has been reported. Cardiac function may improve substantially after treatment with a GFD.

Inflammatory bowel disease. Crohn's disease and ulcerative colitis are more common in people with celiac disease than in the general population, and symptoms of these conditions may be misattributed to celiac disease in relapse. Bowel radiology and colonoscopy with biopsies should clarify the diagnosis.

Other autoimmune diseases such as Sjögren's syndrome, Addison's disease, primary hyperparathyroidism, hypoparathyroidism, hypopituitarism, rheumatoid arthritis, systemic lupus erythematosus, dermatomyositis and immune thrombocytopenic purpura occur with celiac disease, but these have usually been described in small series or as single case reports.

Other associated diseases

The prevalence of celiac disease is increased in some genetic disorders, particularly Down, Turner and Williams syndromes; around 5% of individuals with Down syndrome are affected with celiac disease. Symptoms are often mild and the diagnosis is delayed if systematic screening is not performed. Anti-gliadin antibody (AGA) of both immunoglobulin (Ig)A and IgG classes can be found in many individuals with Down syndrome but not celiac disease. Although patients may have joint disturbances is it is not clear whether specific disorders occur in celiac disease. There may also be an association with cystic fibrosis and tuberculosis.

Patients with selective IgA deficiency (serum IgA < 5 mg/dL) have a 10–15-fold increased risk of developing celiac disease.

Gluten neuropathy

In 1996, investigators from Sheffield, England, reported gluten sensitivity based on the presence of AGA in patients with neurological disorders of unknown cause; duodenal biopsy revealed celiac disease to be present in only one-third of this group. The terms 'gluten neuropathy' and 'gluten ataxia' were coined to describe these disorders. The clinical and immunologic features of 100 patients in this group are shown in Table 4.4.

Some patients with gluten ataxia improve when given a GFD, even in the absence of an enteropathy. The evidence supporting gluten ataxia as an entity is strong and based on findings such as the presence of circulating AGA, the association with HLA-DQ2, the presence of circulating Purkinje cell antibody, the presence of anti-tissue transglutaminase antibody (anti-tTG) in the gut and brain and clinical improvement on a GFD. This work extends even further the concept of gluten sensitivity beyond the bowel (celiac disease) and the skin (dermatitis herpetiformis) to involve the nervous system.

TABLE 4.4

Clinical and immunologic features of 100 patients with gluten neuropathy

Feature	Proportion of individuals with feature (%)
Sensorimotor axonal neuropathy	67
Mononeuropathy multiplex	17
Motor neuropathy	9
Small-fiber neuropathy	7
Only IgG AGA	57
Only IgA AGA	16
Both IgA and IgG AGA	27
IgA class anti-tTG	36 (16/44)
IgA class AEA	23 (12/52)
Enteropathy on duodenal biopsy	29 (26/89)
HLA of celiac disease	80 (80/100)

AEA, anti-endomysial antibody; AGA, anti-gliadin antibody; HLA, human leukocyte antigen; IgA/G, immunoglobulin A/G; anti-tTG, anti-tissue transglutaminase antibody.
Data from Hadjivassiliou et al., 2006.

Dermatitis herpetiformis

Dermatitis herpetiformis is part of the spectrum of celiac disease and is discussed in Chapter 7.

Failure to respond to a gluten-free diet

The concept of non-responsive celiac disease has generated much debate. If celiac disease is defined as a condition that responds to a GFD in terms of symptoms and the morphology of the small-bowel mucosa then, by definition, celiac disease is not present if there is no response. If, however, a less restrictive definition is used and the criterion for diagnosis is a flat mucosa, irrespective of the response to a GFD, then non-responsiveness can be accepted. In any event, 10–15% of patients continue to have symptoms on a GFD and require assessment, while

others may respond symptomatically to diet, but still have a flat
or severely damaged mucosa. The first requirement is to check the
strictness of the GFD. The commonest cause for poor response is that
patients are taking gluten deliberately or inadvertently and this should
be checked by a dietician with a detailed knowledge of the diet.
Serological tests and repeat small-bowel biopsies will help in the
assessment.

Non-response can be classified as clinical or histological. Clinical
non-response manifests as persistence of symptoms or return of
symptoms while on a strict GFD. The small-bowel mucosa is normal
because the conditions causing it are not directly related to celiac
disease (Table 4.5). Histological non-response may also be primary
or secondary and symptoms are usually present.

A number of the conditions listed in Table 4.5 are amenable to
treatment, but some patients do not improve and are regarded as having
refractory celiac disease. This may be defined as persisting villous
atrophy with crypt hyperplasia in those who have taken a strict GFD

TABLE 4.5

Causes of clinical and histological non-response to a gluten-free diet

Clinical non-response

- Pancreatic insufficiency
- Secondary lactase deficiency
- Collagenous colitis
- Lymphocytic colitis
- Bacterial overgrowth in the small bowel
- Inflammatory bowel disease
  - Ulcerative colitis
  - Crohn's disease
- Irritable bowel syndrome

Histological non-response

- Other food intolerances (e.g. milk, egg, chicken, tuna, soy)
- Trace element deficiencies (e.g. zinc)
- Intestinal lymphoma
- Small-intestinal carcinoma
- Ulcerative jejunoileitis
- Mesenteric lymph node cavitation
- Collagenous sprue

for more than 12 months or, when severe symptoms necessitate, other interventions. Many of these patients will have chronic ulcerative jejunoileitis, which falls within the spectrum of small-bowel lymphoma, and therefore have a poor outlook (see Chapter 8).

There are a few rare conditions with villous atrophy not related to celiac disease, such as autoimmune enteropathy, small-bowel clonal T-cell proliferation, chronic idiopathic enterocolitis and common variable immunodeficiency. Initially, these may be confused with celiac disease, but measurement of antibodies associated with celiac disease and determination of the HLA status will help to make the differentiation. These conditions will not respond to a GFD.

Key points – clinical manifestations

- Celiac disease presents with a wide spectrum of clinical manifestations in children and adults, and the diagnosis is easily missed if it is not actively considered.
- Typical manifestations of celiac disease in young children include chronic diarrhea, weight loss, poor appetite and abdominal distension.
- Of adults with the disease, 25% are now diagnosed over the age of 60 years and 10% over the age of 70 years.
- Only about half of adults present with diarrhea. Many complain of mild or non-specific complaints such as lethargy, poor appetite, weight loss and abdominal bloating.
- Autoimmune diseases coexist with celiac disease, the commonest being type 1 diabetes mellitus and thyroid disorders.
- Failure to respond to a GFD indicates the presence of a second diagnosis or that a serious complication has arisen, such as intestinal lymphoma or ulcerative jejunoileitis.

Key references

Bonamico M, Mariani P, Danesi HM et al. Prevalence and clinical picture of celiac disease in Italian Down syndrome patients: a multicenter study. *J Pediatr Gastroenterol Nutr* 2001;33:139–43.

Catassi C, Kryszak D, Louis-Jacques O et al. Detection of celiac disease in primary care: a multicenter case-finding study in North America. *Am J Gastroenterol* 2007;102:1454–60.

Elfström P, Montgomery SM, Kämpe O et al. Risk of thyroid disease in individuals with celiac disease. *J Clin Endocrinol Metab* 2008;93:3915–21.

Fasano A, Catassi C. Coeliac disease in children. *Best Pract Res Clin Gastroenterol* 2005;19:467–78.

Gobbi G. Coeliac disease, epilepsy and cerebral calcifications. *Brain Dev* 2005;27:189–200.

Hadjivassiliou M, Grünewald RA, Kandler RH et al. Neuropathy associated with gluten sensitivity. *J Neurol Neurosurg Psychiatry* 2006;77:1262–6.

Holmes GKT. Coeliac disease and Type 1 diabetes mellitus – the case for screening. *Diabet Med* 2001;18: 169–77.

Holmes GKT. Screening for coeliac disease in type 1 diabetes. *Arch Dis Child* 2002;87:495–8.

Rubio-Tapia A, Murray JA. The liver in celiac disease. *Hepatology* 2007;46:1650–8.

West J, Logan RFA, Hill PG et al. Seroprevalence, correlates, and characteristics of undetected coeliac disease in England. *Gut* 2003;52: 960–5.

Increasing understanding of the presentations of celiac disease, the varied appearances of small-bowel biopsies and the advent of reliable serological tests have forced changes in the criteria for diagnosis and these will continue to evolve. A high index of clinical suspicion is essential to identify patients with celiac disease. Once the possibility has been recognized, tests should be carried out to confirm the diagnosis (Table 5.1). Making the diagnosis of celiac disease is like trying to solve a puzzle by collecting and correctly interpreting pieces of evidence – clinical, serological, histological and genetic. This process is straightforward in most cases, but difficult scenarios continue to arise in clinical practice. If complications of malignancy or bowel ulceration are suspected at presentation, additional investigations will be required.

Routine blood tests

Hematologic and biochemical profiles should be obtained for all patients whenever possible.

Anemia is often present and should not be overlooked, even when it is mild. Measurement of serum ferritin, folate and vitamin B_{12} will help to

---

TABLE 5.1

Tests to confirm a diagnosis of celiac disease

- Routine blood tests and the measurement of specific indices
- Serological markers
- HLA markers
- Biopsy of small-intestinal mucosa
- Tests of intestinal absorption
- Imaging

HLA, human leukocyte antigen.

establish the cause of the anemia. Folate and ferritin deficiencies are common and, while low concentrations of vitamin B_{12} are often found, pernicious anemia is rare in celiac disease.

Mean corpuscular volume. A low or elevated mean corpuscular volume (MCV) sometimes occurs in the absence of anemia and reflects deficiencies of iron (low MCV), and of folate and vitamin B_{12} (high MCV).

Features of hyposplenism (e.g. Howell-Jolly bodies, thrombocytosis) are most commonly caused by celiac disease if the patient has not had a splenectomy.

Pancytopenia is uncommon and is usually due to folate or vitamin B_{12} deficiency.

A prolonged prothrombin time caused by vitamin K deficiency is rare, but should be corrected before taking a small-bowel biopsy.

Lymphocytopenia may be present and probably reflects the lymphoid atrophy associated with celiac disease.

Hypocalcemia, hypophosphatemia and elevated alkaline phosphatase indicate osteomalacia. Hypocalcemia may, however, occur as an isolated finding.

Aminotransferases (aspartate and alanine) may be mildly elevated in celiac disease.

Mild hypoalbuminemia may be present, and may reflect increased protein loss in the gut and reduced liver synthesis. Marked hypoalbuminemia indicates severe malabsorption or the presence of complications such as lymphoma or bowel ulcerations.

IgA deficiency. Celiac disease is ten times more common in individuals deficient in immunoglobulin (Ig)A than in the general population.

Serological markers of celiac disease

Reliable serological investigations have a place:

- if the probability of celiac disease is low, as a negative antibody test will avoid a biopsy
- when identifying cases in groups at particular risk of celiac disease (e.g. relatives of patients with celiac disease, patients with type 1 diabetes mellitus)
- in monitoring compliance with a gluten-free diet (GFD)
- when high levels of anti-tissue transglutaminase antibodies (anti-tTG) in patients who are usually symptomatic are accepted as being diagnostic of celiac disease, so that small-bowel biopsies are not considered necessary.

IgA and IgG anti-gliadin antibodies (AGA), introduced in the early 1980s, were the first serological markers of celiac disease to be widely used in clinical practice; IgA-class AGA is more specific and IgG AGA is more sensitive for celiac disease. Other tests with better sensitivity and specificity (Table 5.2) have taken their place, though they have a role in the diagnosis of gluten ataxia (see pages 52–3).

If gliadin gains access to the immune system through 'leaky' mucous membranes, antibodies will be produced so raised levels may also be found in a number of other conditions, such as esophagitis, gastritis,

TABLE 5.2

Sensitivities and specificities of IgA-class antibody tests for detecting celiac disease

IgA antibody	Sensitivity (%)	Specificity (%)
ARA	35–75	95
AGA*	58–75	80–95
AEA	95	99
Anti-tTG	95	99

*First-generation test.
AEA, anti-endomysial antibody; AGA, anti-gliadin antibody; ARA, anti-reticulin antibody; anti-tTG, anti-tissue transglutaminase antibody; IgA, immunoglobulin A.

recent gastroenteritis, ulcerative colitis and Crohn's disease. Anti-endomysial (AEA) and anti-tTG are not detected in these disorders.

A second-generation AGA test using deamidated gliadin as the antigen has been recently developed. This test, particularly the IgG component, seems to have a specificity as high as that of IgA anti-tTG.

IgA anti-reticulin antibody (ARA) reacts against extracellular connective tissue fibrils (reticulin). It is detected by indirect immunofluorescence using rodent tissue (i.e. serum samples are incubated with tissue sections such as liver, antibodies bind to the tissue and are detected using immunofluorescence); the test is included by some laboratories as part of a general autoimmune screening profile. ARA positivity is, therefore, often an opportunistic finding and should lead to more specific testing for celiac disease.

IgA anti-endomysial antibody is an autoantibody directed against antigens in the collagenous matrix of human and monkey tissues. AEA is produced by biopsies from untreated celiac patients and from treated patients challenged in vitro with gliadin. The usual method for detecting IgA AEA is indirect immunofluorescence with sections of either monkey esophagus or human umbilical cord (Figure 5.1). False-negative results can occur for children under 2 years of age.

The nature of this test renders it more time-consuming to perform, generally more expensive and, because the interpretation is operator dependent, potentially prone to more errors.

Anti-tissue transglutaminase antibody. The enzyme tTG is the major autoantigen responsible for AEA positivity in celiac disease. IgA-class anti-tTG measurement with human recombinant tTG or human-derived red blood cells as the antigen is easily automated and quantitative, unlike AEA detection. This should be the first-line test for detecting celiac disease in children and adults. There are many kits on the market and not all perform to the same high analytical standard. Anti-tTG testing can also be used to monitor compliance with a GFD, but kits vary in the ability to detect an early response to gluten withdrawal.

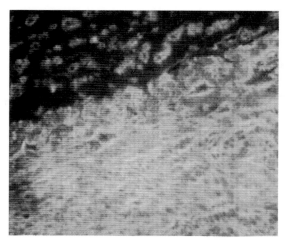

Figure 5.1 Indirect immunofluorescence staining pattern for anti-endomysial antibody using human umbilical cord exposed to serum from a patient with untreated celiac disease. The positivity is seen around the smooth muscle fibers of the vessels as a honeycomb reticular network.

Point-of-care tests using the principles shown in Figure 5.2 are available. They can provide a rapid result for screening purposes.

IgA anti-actin antibody. Actin is a key structural protein of the cytoskeletal network, and is particularly abundant in intestinal microvilli. IgA-class anti-actin antibody, detectable in the sera of celiac patients using immunofluorescence or enzyme-linked immunosorbent assay, has recently been suggested as a marker of severe intestinal villous atrophy.

False-positive and false-negative antibody results

False-positive anti-tTG results may occur in conditions where serum Ig concentrations are raised, such as chronic liver disease with raised polyclonal IgA and in myeloma with high monoclonal IgA levels. In these cases the anti-tTG titer is rarely more than five times the upper limit of normal and the AEA result is negative. A duodenal biopsy is unnecessary in these patients unless clinical considerations dictate otherwise. A positive test may be found in patients with normal or near-normal histology on small-bowel biopsy. These patients are

61

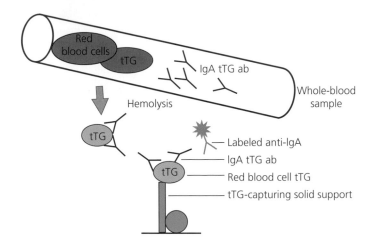

Figure 5.2 Principle of measuring anti-tissue transglutaminase antibody (anti-tTG) IgA from a whole-blood sample using an in-house point-of-care test. First, the celiac autoantigen tTG is liberated from red blood cells by hemolyzing the whole-blood sample. Anti-tTG present in the serum forms complexes with liberated tTG. The formed complexes are bound to a solid surface with the help of tTG/fibronectin-capture proteins. The IgA-class anti-tTG antibody of the complexes is visualized in a color reaction by labeled anti-human IgA.

regarded as having potential celiac disease and their symptoms, if any, may respond to a GFD. In due course they may develop villous atrophy.

AEA and anti-tTG tests have about 95% sensitivity, so some patients will have small-bowel biopsies characteristic of celiac disease but negative tests. A biopsy should always be carried out if, on clinical grounds, celiac disease is suspected but the serological tests are negative. The response to a GFD or gluten challenge will help to clarify the diagnosis but these approaches are time-consuming and laborious. It should not be forgotten that a flat biopsy is found in autoimmune enteropathy, a condition associated with anti-enterocyte antibody but negative serological tests for celiac disease and no response to a GFD.

The absence of HLA-DQ2 and HLA-DQ8 rules out a diagnosis of celiac disease with 99% confidence.

Selective IgA deficiency

An associated selective IgA deficiency occurs in 2–3% of celiac patients, representing at least a tenfold increase over the prevalence in the general population. IgA antibodies are not generated by IgA-deficient individuals, so a testing strategy must ensure that the diagnosis is not missed in these patients. When measuring anti-tTG, total serum IgA measurement is required only in the small proportion of samples that produce a result at the lower end of the reference range. This strategy will reduce the need to measure IgA by about 90% depending on the kit used. If AEA is used as a first-line test, IgA should be measured in all cases. If selective IgA deficiency is established, then IgG-class anti-tTG should be measured.

HLA-DQ2 and HLA-DQ8

About 90% of patients with celiac disease have HLA-DQ2 and about 5% are HLA-DQ8 positive. The few patients who do not belong to these categories usually carry one of the two chains of the DQ2 heterodimer ('half' DQ2), most frequently the DQB1*02 allele. These markers are also present in 30–40% of Caucasian populations, so they are only useful in a negative sense, celiac disease being effectively ruled out in their absence. The HLA test is of value in excluding the diagnosis in those who have, for example, type 1 diabetes or a family risk, where periodic screening for celiac disease is required.

Biopsy of small-intestinal mucosa

The diagnosis of celiac disease has centered on the appearance of the jejunal mucosa and the responses to gluten withdrawal and challenge and associated clinical reactions. As understanding has increased, the concept of silent, latent and potential celiac disease has emerged, which, together with the development of serological tests, is forcing re-evaluation of the diagnostic criteria. Biopsy of the small intestine is, however, still considered the cornerstone of diagnosis.

Obtaining biopsies. Biopsies can be taken using a capsule with a suction-guillotine mechanism (e.g. Crosby capsule, Watson capsule). Nowadays, most biopsies are taken at the time of upper gastrointestinal endoscopy using standard fiber-optic instruments.

Upper gastrointestinal endoscopy is safe, quick and accurate; although uncomfortable, it is not painful so patients can be reassured that it is not as daunting as it sounds. Before endoscopy, patients should not take any fluids by mouth for 2 hours or food for 4 hours. Essential medications are allowed. When the patient is lying in the left lateral position on the table in the endoscopy room the back of the throat is sprayed with a local anesthetic and a mouth guard is inserted between the teeth to protect the delicate endoscope. Intravenous sedation is available for those who are particularly anxious but most decide not to have it. Individuals who elect to have sedation should be accompanied and should not drive or operate machinery for at least 12 hours. In children, the procedure is carried out under a general anesthetic. The endoscope is then passed over the tongue and into the esophagus, stomach and duodenum with air insufflation so that good views of the lumen can be obtained. When the endoscope is in the second part of the duodenum, 3–6 biopsies are taken of the mucosa, which will support or refute the diagnosis of celiac disease. As the endoscope is withdrawn, air is removed to make the patient more comfortable. The procedure takes 5–10 minutes. Afterwards, a doctor or nurse will review the patient; the views provided by endoscopy may enable a confidant diagnosis of celiac disease at that time, but a definitive diagnosis must await the biopsy results, which will be available after about a week. Once the diagnosis is certain, the patient can be seen with a view to commencing a GFD.

Endoscopy allows multiple biopsies to be taken, which minimizes sampling error; in many patients, views of the mucosa will support or refute the diagnosis even before the results of the biopsies are available. Biopsies are small, but some pathologists like the samples to be oriented before fixation on a cellulose strip with the villi uppermost, in order to make a correct evaluation. Others consider that attempts to orient the samples may result in damage and prefer the specimens to be placed floating free in formalin. High-resolution magnification endoscopy is a further aid to diagnosis and may help to identify areas particularly suitable for biopsy.

Enteroscopy offers the opportunity to take mucosal biopsies further down the small bowel. It also allows inspection for other pathologies such as ulcerations, lymphomas and carcinomas, which can also be biopsied. The procedure can be uncomfortable and can cause respiratory difficulties. It also carries the risk of intestinal perforation.

Biopsy capsules retrieve larger biopsies that can be oriented and placed on card to be inspected under the dissecting microscope, which will differentiate normal from flat specimens. These devices are now very seldom used in routine clinical practice.

Histological evaluation

In routine practice the diagnosis is based on morphologic appearances after the tissue is fixed, sectioned and stained with hematoxylin and eosin (Figure 5.3). When appearances are not straightforward, the villus–crypt ratio can be measured (normal ≥ 3), intraepithelial lymphocyte (IEL) counts performed (normal < 25 per 100 enterocytes), and CD3 and CD8 markers employed. The last of these are particularly helpful if enteropathy-associated T-cell lymphoma is suspected. In those with normal or near-normal mucosa (type 1 lesion), the detection of subepithelial tTG-2-specific IgA deposits by immunochemistry on frozen samples is predictive of villous atrophy (see Figure 1.2, page 10).

Tests of intestinal absorption

Fecal fat measurement. Steatorrhea can be shown by microscopy. As many patients do not have steatorrhea and better tests are available, the measurement of fat is now obsolete and has no part to play in the diagnosis of celiac disease.

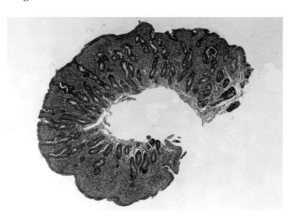

Figure 5.3 Biopsy of the duodenum in celiac disease taken at endoscopy.

Intestinal permeability. The permeability of the intestinal mucosa can be assessed using differential sugar absorption. This test is performed by measuring the urinary recovery, after oral administration, of two sugars of different molecular sizes and different absorption routes, such as lactulose and mannitol (Figure 5.4). A usual finding in untreated celiac disease is increased urinary excretion of lactulose (due to increased paracellular enterocyte permeability) associated with decreased mannitol recovery (because of reduced intestinal mucosal surface) (see Figure 3.10, page 33). It should be noted, however, that the results can be normal in some patients with either atypical or silent

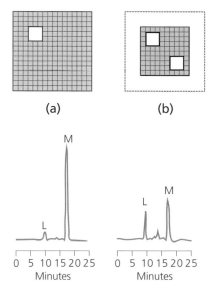

(a)   (b)

Figure 5.4 The intestinal permeability test. The monosaccharide (mannitol) crosses the mucosa through water-filled intracellular pores (small squares), while the disaccharide (lactulose) is larger and can permeate only through the intercellular junctions (large squares). (a) Normal mucosa and its high-performance liquid chromatography pattern of urinary recovery of permeability probes. (b) When the mucosa is damaged the number of water-filled pores decreases because of the reduction in absorptive surface, while intercellular permeation increases. This is reflected by a decreased recovery of mannitol and increased recovery of lactulose in the urine. M, mannitol; L, lactulose.

celiac disease, probably because the mucosal damage extends only a short way down the bowel. In practice, the permeability test offers no advantages over serological tests.

Imaging

Bowel radiology. Dilatation of the small bowel with thickening of the mucosal folds and clumping of the barium are features seen on follow-through examination (Figure 5.5). It is not necessary to perform bowel radiology routinely, but it should be considered if:

- patients are unusually ill at presentation, with dramatic weight loss, abdominal pain, features of intestinal obstruction or abdominal masses
- blood tests show marked abnormalities (e.g. severe anemia, low albumin)
- occult blood loss is found
- newly diagnosed patients do not show the expected responses to a GFD or response is lost in established cases.

Under these circumstances, ulcerative jejunoileitis or small-bowel lymphoma or carcinoma may be present.

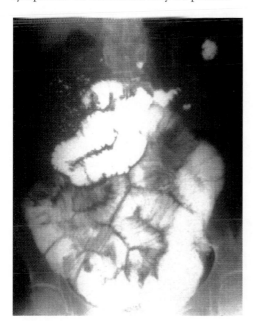

Figure 5.5 Appearance of the small bowel in untreated celiac disease on barium follow-through examination, showing dilatation of the bowel and coarsening of the valvulae.

Scanning. Ultrasound, computed tomography (CT) and magnetic resonance imaging (MRI) may be helpful in patients who are severely ill at presentation, who do not show the expected responses to gluten withdrawal and in those in whom the response is lost. Enlarged lymph nodes denoting lymphoma or mesenteric lymph-node cavitation syndrome may be found (Figure 5.6). Abdominal bowel sonography is now very widely carried out for many indications, and awareness of the findings indicating celiac disease is important. These include:

- fluid-filled bowel loops
- increased peristalsis
- thickened valvulae conniventes
- intussusception
- free fluid in the abdomen.

Capsule endoscopy is having an increasingly important role in the investigation of small-bowel disease to establish, for example, the cause of obscure intestinal bleeding and the diagnosis of Crohn's disease in difficult cases. While it would not be used as a first-line test to diagnose celiac disease, operators need to be aware of appearances indicative of celiac disease. There is also a role in those suspected of having developed complications of celiac disease.

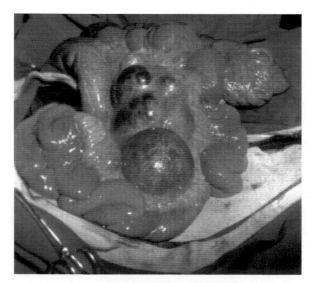

Figure 5.6
Mesentery of the small bowel in a patient with celiac disease showing large cavitating lymph nodes.

Gluten challenge

Gluten challenge is a provocation test performed to confirm the diagnosis of celiac disease and is used only when there are doubts about the initial diagnosis. After the patient has been treated with a GFD for at least 12–24 months, gluten is re-introduced through free intake of gluten-containing products. A further small-bowel biopsy is performed either when symptoms of relapse appear or after 6–24 months. Deterioration of the mucosal architecture confirms the persistence of gluten intolerance and the patient is returned to a GFD.

In adults, gluten challenge has very little place. It is used occasionally to confirm the diagnosis in patients who started a GFD before a biopsy was taken. A biopsy should be obtained after 3–6 months on a normal diet or earlier if symptoms occur.

Diagnosis in children

In most children the diagnosis is strengthened by positive celiac serology (IgA anti-tTG and AEA) and is confirmed by finding celiac enteropathy at small-bowel biopsy. The small-intestinal biopsy is considered the gold standard for diagnosis, but this is likely to change in the near future because of the excellent sensitivity and the specificity of serological tests. A quantitative approach to the diagnosis of celiac disease in children is proposed that employs the '4 out of 5' rule, i.e. the diagnosis of celiac disease is confirmed when at least 4 out of 5 criteria are met (Table 5.3). The application of this scheme overcomes difficulties with current algorithms (e.g. in patients with potential celiac disease), or lack of HLA-DQ2 and -DQ8 (as may exceptionally happen), or in young sick children whose parents refuse the small-intestinal biopsy. It is important to underline that a gluten challenge after a GFD is always indicated whenever there are doubts about the initial diagnosis.

Diagnosis in adults

For patients in the Western world, a flat biopsy from the small intestine almost certainly indicates celiac disease, and many would accept the diagnosis based on this criterion. Some require a clinical response to gluten withdrawal to make the diagnosis, but this cannot be used in those who do not have symptoms. Others require demonstration of

TABLE 5.3

Criteria for the diagnosis of celiac disease in children

The diagnosis is confirmed when 4 out of 5 of the following criteria are met:

- Typical presentation, including failure to thrive
- Positivity of celiac serology (high-titer anti-tTG and AEA)
- Celiac enteropathy on small-bowel biopsy (grades 1–3)
- HLA-DQ2 and/or -DQ8
- Response to a gluten-free diet

AEA, anti-endomysial antibody; anti-tTG, anti-tissue transglutaminase antibody; HLA, human leukocyte antigen.

an improvement in the appearances of the mucosa; in practice, while continuing abnormality may indicate laxity with the GFD, it seldom changes the diagnosis.

How the diagnosis should be established in adults is in a state of flux. An initial biopsy is still considered mandatory by many, but the advent of reliable serological tests is increasingly challenging this view, as it is in pediatric practice. More and more, doctors faced with patients who are usually symptomatic with high anti-tTG levels are questioning whether a biopsy is necessary, as indeed are patients themselves. At least 10% of biopsies are of such poor quality that they cannot be used in the diagnostic process and mild histological changes can be impossible to interpret.

A study from Derby, UK, has shown that it is possible to define an anti-tTG level which gives a positive predictive value for celiac disease of 100% and removes the requirement for duodenal biopsy completely in over half of patients. Such observations will challenge the necessity of small-intestinal biopsy to establish the diagnosis of celiac disease and force modification of guidelines.

Key points – diagnosis

- A high index of suspicion is essential to identify patients with celiac disease.
- Anti-tissue transglutaminase antibody measurement should be the first-line serological test because it has many analytical advantages over the anti-endomysial antibody assay.
- A small-bowel biopsy is still regarded by many as mandatory, but the availability of reliable quantitative serological tests is increasingly challenging this view.
- Lack or loss of response to a gluten-free diet may indicate the development of a complication and requires urgent investigation.

Key references

Fernández E, Blanco C, García S et al. Use of low concentrations of human IgA anti-tissue transglutaminase to rule out selective IgA deficiency in patients with suspected celiac disease. *Clin Chem* 2005;51:1014–16.

Hill PG, Holmes GKT. Coeliac disease; a biopsy is not always necessary for diagnosis. *Aliment Pharmacol Ther* 2008;27:572–7.

Hill PG, McMillan SA. Anti-tissue transglutaminase antibodies and their role in the investigation of coeliac disease. *Ann Clin Biochem* 2006;43:105–17.

Hopper AD, Cross SS, Hurlstone DP et al. Pre-endoscopy serological testing for coeliac disease: evaluation of a clinical decision tool. *BMJ* 2007;334:729.

Korponay-Szabó IR, Szabados K, Pusztai J et al. Population screening for coeliac disease in primary care by district nurses using a rapid antibody test: diagnostic accuracy and feasibility study. *BMJ* 2007;335:1244–7.

Rashtak S, Ettore MW, Homburger HA, Murray JA. Comparative usefulness of deamidated gliadin antibodies in the diagnosis of celiac disease. *Clin Gastroenterol Hepatol* 2008;6:426–32.

Non-malignant complications of celiac disease can be troublesome and even life-threatening. Prevention is better than cure and it is important that patients are diagnosed before complications occur, because a gluten-free diet (GFD) may prevent them or reduce the risks of development.

Disorders of bone and calcium metabolism

Celiac disease predisposes to abnormalities of bone and calcium metabolism, which result in rickets, osteomalacia and osteoporosis. Techniques that allow the accurate measurement of bone mineral density, parathyroid hormone concentrations, vitamin D metabolites and markers of bone formation and resorption provide means of exploring these facets of celiac disease.

Pathogenesis. The pathogenesis of osteopenia is not fully understood, but the development of hypocalcemia is likely to be the central event that leads to parathyroid hormone release and bone resorption. A number of mechanisms lead to hypocalcemia (Table 6.1).

TABLE 6.1

Mechanisms leading to hypocalcemia

- A reduced intake of calcium
- Associated lactose intolerance restricting milk and therefore calcium intake
- Increased endogenous loss
- Loss of surface area for absorption
- Low concentration of 25-hydroxycolecalciferol
- Reduced responsiveness of the small bowel to 1,25-dihydroxycolecalciferol promoting malabsorption of calcium
- Reduction of calcium transport proteins (e.g. calbindin)

Increased concentrations of 1,25-dihydroxycolecalciferol are found in patients taking a normal diet because the enzyme 1α-hydroxylase is enhanced. The levels fall in those following a GFD, but may remain above normal, possibly accounting for the incomplete recovery of bone mass observed in some treated patients. A GFD also tends to normalize parathyroid hormone and serum calcium. The markers of bone remodeling, osteocalcin and serum carboxy-terminal propeptide of type 1 procollagen (markers of formation), and serum carboxy-terminal pyridinolone crosslinked telopeptide of type 1 collagen (a marker of resorption), are significantly increased in untreated compared with treated patients and indicate increased bone turnover. Malabsorption of vitamin D results in rickets and osteomalacia.

Clinical features and diagnosis. The severe clinical forms of osteomalacia are now rarely seen and the present challenge is to detect those patients who have no or only minor symptoms of celiac or bone disease. Early recognition and treatment will prevent more severe problems arising. Osteomalacia can occur in the absence of gastrointestinal symptoms or steatorrhea, and may be the presenting complaint. Myopathy may be a prominent presenting feature of osteomalacia in celiac patients. Fracture is the only cause of symptoms in osteoporosis. Vertebral fractures present with the sudden onset of quite severe pain. However, two-thirds of these fractures present only with height loss and kyphosis. Breaks of the neck of the femur and Colles' fractures are common and typically occur as a result of falls, particularly in the elderly. A common presentation is with radiological osteopenia on X-ray examination for trauma or other reasons.

Routine biochemical profiles, which include calcium, phosphate and alkaline phosphatase assays, may indicate the presence of osteomalacia, but osteomalacia can be present even if these indices are normal. 25-hydroxyvitamin D may be measured. Elevated parathyroid hormone in the presence of a normal serum calcium result indicates secondary hyperparathyroidism, which can be treated. Bone biopsy may be undertaken, but is not usually necessary. Monitoring the response to a GFD and vitamin D by symptoms, if present, and changes in the blood chemistry may be sufficient.

Blood tests in the diagnosis of osteoporosis are unhelpful, but bone mineral density can be reliably measured by dual-energy X-ray absorptiometry (DEXA) (see Figure 4.4, page 44). Results are expressed as the number of standard deviations (SDs) above or below the mean value for young adults (T-score) or age-matched controls (Z-score). Osteoporosis is defined as a T-score equal to or below 2.5, while a value between −1 and −2.5 is regarded as osteopenia, which, in due course, may lead to osteoporosis (see *Fast Facts: Osteoporosis*). There is a moderate reduction in bone mineral density in untreated celiac disease which improves significantly on a GFD. Fracture risk increases 1.4–2.6 times for each SD decrease in bone mineral density. The fracture risk in celiac disease is about 1.4 for all fractures.

The modest increase in risk of fracture and bone mineral density cannot justify performing DEXA in all patients. Whether to carry out DEXA will depend on the presence of:
- risk factors of patients (Table 6.2)
- radiological evidence of osteopenia
- classic symptoms of celiac disease
- poor adherence to the GFD.

TABLE 6.2

Risk factors for the development of osteoporosis

- Advancing age
- Female sex
- Caucasian or Asian race
- Family history of osteoporosis
- Hypogonadism
- Steroid therapy
- Low body mass index
- Previous fragility fracture

- Associated disorders including
  - celiac disease
  - hyperthyroidism
  - hyperparathyroidism
  - Crohn's disease
  - liver disease
  - renal disease
- Immobilization
- Cigarette smoking
- Excessive alcohol intake

There is no point in ordering a DEXA scan for those without risk factors who are well on a GFD.

The best time to carry out a scan is debatable. In individuals with risk factors, we suggest that a scan be performed when the diagnosis of celiac disease is made. After 1–2 years of dietary management (with a GFD) and treatment for osteoporosis the scan should be repeated to monitor progress.

Treatment. Some of the many risk factors for osteoporosis in celiac disease can be modified and this offers an opportunity to reduce the fracture risk. To address the obvious ones, patients should be advised to:

• keep active
• take a nutritious diet with adequate calcium and, if necessary, calcium supplements to ensure an intake of 1500 mg per day
• maintain a healthy body weight
• stop smoking
• avoid excess alcohol consumption.

Apart from any other considerations these are sensible measures to take for healthy living. Risk factors for falling are also major determinants of a fracture occurring, particularly fractures of the hip in the elderly (Table 6.3). Some of these can also be modified to reduce the fracture risk.

Specific measures. The aim is to restore the small-intestinal mucosa to normal by adopting a GFD, so that the mechanisms which promote absorption of calcium and vitamin D can become fully effective. Improvements in bone scores can be detected within 1 year of beginning a GFD and the bones may return to normal after 4–10 years. In children and adolescents, a GFD alone can restore bone density. In adults, other treatments such as calcium supplements, vitamin D, hormone replacement and bisphosphonates may be required.

Osteomalacia will be reversed by vitamin D, calcium supplements and a GFD.

Splenic atrophy and hyposplenism

Hyposplenism assessed by pitted red cell counts occurs in adult celiac patients but not in children. A prevalence of 80% is found in those with

TABLE 6.3

Risk factors for fracture other than bone mineral density

- Poor visual acuity
- Cognitive impairment
- Reduced mobility
- Neuromuscular weakness
- Incoordination
- Use of sedatives and tranquilizers
- Use of alcohol
- Environmental hazards e.g. uneven floors, loose carpets, poor lighting
- Ill-fitting or inappropriate footwear

complicated celiac disease (lymphoma, refractory celiac disease or ulcerative jejunoileitis), 60% in those with other associated autoimmune disorders and 20% in uncomplicated disease. This defect may predispose to sepsis and an increased risk has been demonstrated, particularly for pneumococcal infection. Those who appear at greatest risk should be considered for vaccination with a conjugate pneumococcal vaccine.

Neurological and psychiatric disorders

Epidemiology. The true prevalence of neurological and psychiatric complications in celiac disease is difficult to estimate because of differences in study criteria and varying definitions of neurological disorder. Moreover, most prevalence analyses have been performed in selected patient groups in tertiary referral centers, which skews the figures. It has been estimated that about 10% of patients with celiac disease develop neurological complications, but this is almost certainly an underestimate. Data from one celiac clinic in Derby, England, which is not a referral center, found 160 neurological and 103 psychiatric conditions in 620 patients (some had more than one disorder) (Table 6.4). Which disorders, if any, are specific for celiac disease is unknown.

TABLE 6.4

Commonest neurological and psychiatric complications found in 620 patients attending the Derby celiac clinic

Disorder	Number of patients affected (%)
Depression	71 (11.5)
Epilepsy	25 (4.0)
Migraine	20 (3.2)
Carpal tunnel syndrome	15 (2.4)
Stroke	15 (2.4)
Anxiety	13 (2.1)
Self-poisoning	11 (1.8)
Myopathy	8 (1.3)
Learning difficulty	7 (1.1)
Sciatica	6 (1.0)
Meningitis	5 (0.8)
Parkinson's disease	4 (0.6)
Tension headache	4 (0.6)
Multiple sclerosis	3 (0.5)
Peripheral neuropathy	3 (0.5)
Ataxia	2 (0.3)

The commonest problem is depression. It can be so severe that patients may attempt and succeed in committing suicide. Epilepsy occurs and there is an association between celiac disease, epilepsy and intracranial calcifications (Figure 6.1), though why these phenomena should be present together is not understood. The geographic distribution of these patients is also puzzling, as most have occurred in Italy and none in the UK. Migraine is the third most common condition encountered. Whether these conditions occur more commonly in celiac disease than in the general population is unknown, but seems unlikely. Many other conditions are encountered, but usually as single cases even in large celiac clinics. There are numerous descriptions of spinocerebellar and cerebellar disorders, with frequent reports of

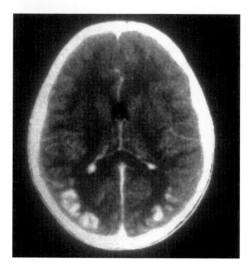

Figure 6.1 MRI scan showing intracranial calcifications in a patient with celiac disease and epilepsy.

ataxia in classic celiac disease where gastrointestinal symptoms were concomitant with or preceded the neurological complications (for gluten ataxia, see also Chapter 4). There is no firm link with schizophrenia, autism, multiple sclerosis or dementia.

Etiology. The etiology of these disorders is unknown, but the following factors should be considered.

Heredity. Some spinocerebellar ataxias are linked to human leukocyte antigen (HLA) loci. It is possible that a subgroup of patients with celiac disease develop problems because of a particular genetic profile.

Infection. Immunologic defects in celiac disease may predispose patients to react abnormally to particular infections that might damage neurological tissue.

Toxins. The small-intestinal mucosa in celiac disease is more permeable than normal and could be permeable to substances that are toxic to neurological structures.

Autoimmunity and inflammatory processes. The immunologic disorder found in celiac disease may provoke autoimmune mechanisms that disturb neurological tissue. Occasionally, steroids can cause a transient improvement in symptoms suggesting that inflammatory processes are being calmed.

Vasculitis has been found in association with seizures in celiac disease and could play a part in other neurological disturbances.

Nutritional deficiencies may play a part in the development of neurological and psychiatric disorders because of overt or occult malabsorption. However, it is likely that deficiencies are not sufficient to account for the onset of these disorders as vitamin replacement is rarely helpful and hypovitaminosis is not always detectable. Moreover, there may be no neurological abnormalities in the presence of profound vitamin deficiency.

Treatment. A GFD will usually improve the general health of patients and restore normal small-bowel absorption. The effect of diet, however, on the various neurological and psychiatric problems ranges from reversal of dysfunction, stabilization of the illness to making no difference. Gluten ataxia (see page 52) may improve, as may epilepsy and peripheral neuropathy. Depression and migraine can, in some cases, be alleviated or overcome by following a GFD.

Vitamin replacement. Vitamin deficiencies should be treated, but replacement overall is of little value. Pyridoxine may improve depression and vitamin E may help in some cases of cerebellar ataxia.

Immunosuppressive therapy. It is inevitable that severely ill patients who are deteriorating will be given a trial of steroids and other immunosuppressants, but in general these are of no value.

Reproductive disorders

Results from the many studies in this area are contradictory but this may be due to differences in study populations (patients and controls) and timing of study. The overall message is that patients may have a reduced reproductive period because of a late menarche and early menopause, infertility and poor obstetric histories that can be improved by following a GFD. Also, some women with infertility, poor obstetric histories including small babies and recurrent abortions may have celiac disease, and their caregivers need to be aware of this. It is important to realize that if bowel symptoms are mild or absent, the diagnosis of celiac disease can easily be missed. A liberal use of screening tests should minimize this problem. Following a GFD and taking folic acid may result in conception and delivery of a normal baby. Men with celiac disease may have reversible infertility. Impotence, hypogonadism and abnormal sperm form and motility may occur.

Ulcerative jejunoileitis

Ulcerative jejunoileitis is discussed in Chapter 8 with regard to the malignant potential. It is characterized by malabsorption, with almost always a flat small-intestinal biopsy and chronic ulcers found mainly in the jejunum and ileum, but rarely in the colon (Figure 6.2).
It is likely that most patients have underlying celiac disease. The development of jejunoileitis may bring a patient with celiac disease to diagnosis or cause deterioration in those previously well controlled on a GFD, as may occur with malignancy. Ulcerative jejunoileitis may be premalignant or even a low-grade malignant condition from the onset.

Symptoms and signs include fever, anorexia, weight loss, dehydration, edema, diarrhea and abdominal pain. Patients with suspected ulcerative jejunoileitis should be admitted to hospital, because deterioration is usually relentless and rapid. Initial treatment consists of rehydration with correction of electrolyte disturbances. Intravenous steroids should be given from the outset. Anemia often requires blood transfusion and deficiencies of folic acid, ferritin and vitamins B_{12}, D and K need to be

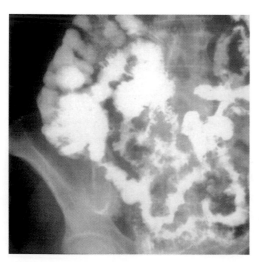

Figure 6.2 Ulcerative jejunoileitis. The small bowel shows a very abnormal pattern with ulceration, thickening of the wall and narrowing of the lumen.

corrected. Malnutrition and hypoalbuminemia are usually marked and require prolonged parenteral feeding. Azathioprine is useful for those not controlled by steroids or needing large doses. Improvement is measured by weight gain and increases in serum albumin concentration. Urgent surgery will be necessary for those who present with intestinal perforation, obstruction or bleeding from the bowel. When enteral feeding becomes possible, a GFD should be given. Milk restriction in the early months may improve symptoms of abdominal bloating, wind and diarrhea. This is a serious complication with a high mortality, but full recovery is possible with intensive support.

Mesenteric lymph node cavitation

Mesenteric lymph node cavitation is a rare serious complication that affects those with long-standing untreated celiac disease and it should also be suspected in patients who do not respond to a GFD (see Figure 5.6, page 68). The condition may be more common than currently thought and it is likely that the increasing use of ultrasound and CT will bring more cases to light. Abdominal masses due to enlarged cystic lymph nodes may be confused with malignant tumors, so an accurate diagnosis is essential. The prognosis is grave, but recovery is possible. Supportive treatments as for ulcerative jejunoileitis are given.

Key points – non-malignant complications

- Individuals with untreated celiac disease demonstrate a modest reduction in bone mineral density and a small increase in fracture risk.
- Many neurological and psychiatric complications occur in celiac disease but it is not known which, if any, are specific or if they are more common in celiac disease than in the general population. The commonest are depression, epilepsy, migraine and ataxia and some may be improved by a gluten-free diet.
- Healthcare professionals need to be aware that women with infertility and poor obstetric histories may have celiac disease and that a gluten-free diet may be helpful.

Key references

Baldwin DS, Hirschfeld KMA. *Fast Facts: Depression*, 2nd edn. Oxford: Health Press, 2005.

Brodie MJ, Schachter SC, Kwan P. *Fast Facts: Epilepsy*, 4th edn. Oxford: Health Press, 2009.

Compston JE, Rosen CJ. *Fast Facts: Osteoporosis*, 6th edn. Oxford: Health Press, 2009.

Di Sabatino A, Rosado MM, Cazzola P et al. Splenic hypofunction and the spectrum of autoimmune and malignant complications in celiac disease. *Clin Gastroenterol Hepatol* 2006;4:179–86.

Greco L, Veneziano A, Di Donato L et al. Undiagnosed coeliac disease does not appear to be associated with unfavourable outcome of pregnancy. *Gut* 2004;53:149–51.

Holmes GKT. Mesenteric lymph node cavitation in coeliac disease. *Gut* 1986;27:728–33.

Holmes GKT. Neurological and psychiatric complications in coeliac disease. In: Gobbi G, Andermann F, Naccarato S, Banchini G, eds. *Epilepsy and Other Neurological Disorders in Coeliac Disease.* London: John Libbey, 1997:251–64.

Lewis NR, Scott BB. Guidelines for osteoporosis in inflammatory bowel disease and coeliac disease. London: British Society of Gastroenterology, 2007.
www.bsg.org.uk/pdf_word_docs/ost_coe_ibd.pdf

Olmos M, Antelo M, Vazquez H et al. Systematic review and meta-analysis of observational studies on the prevalence of fractures in coeliac disease. *Dig Liver Dis* 2008;40:46–53.

Pengiran Tengah DS, Wills AJ, Holmes GKT. Neurological complications of coeliac disease. *Postgrad Med J* 2002;78:393–8.

7   Dermatitis herpetiformis

Dermatitis herpetiformis (DH) was named by Duhring in 1884, though his original description covered several disorders and included conditions such as pemphigoid, pemphigus, herpes gestationis and erythema multiforme. With the development of histological and immunofluorescence techniques and treatments, DH was subsequently shown to be a specific disorder. In 1940, it was observed that the rash was suppressed by sulfapyridine and, 10 years later, dapsone was found to be even more effective.

In the 1960s, two important developments occurred. An enteropathy was found in patients with DH, similar to that found in celiac disease, and immunoglobulin (Ig)A deposits were detected in apparently normal skin, which formed the basis of a diagnostic test.

Epidemiology

DH occurs most commonly in individuals of European origin. The prevalence is approximately 10/100000 in the UK and is the same in the USA among the white population of northern European descent, although higher rates of 40/100000 and 66/100000 have been reported from centers in Sweden and Finland, respectively. DH seldom occurs in Asians and like celiac disease is rare in blacks.

DH can present at any age, but is rare at the extremes of life; the mean age at presentation is about 40 years. In contrast with celiac disease, for which the male to female patient ratio is 1:1.3, DH is more common in men than in women (1.5–1.9:1).

Family studies indicate that 5% of first-degree relatives will also have DH and 5% will have celiac disease; the relatives of patients with these conditions should always be screened. Both conditions have the same prevalence of HLA-DQ2 (90%) and DQ8. Monozygotic twins, of whom one has DH and the other celiac disease, are known. These observations emphasize the link between the two disorders.

Etiology

It is not known why only some patients with celiac disease develop DH and what factors link the bowel and skin lesions. In DH, IgA is present in the skin, and inflammatory cells and cytokines are found in the lesions. Furthermore, anti-endomysial antibody (AEA), anti-tissue transglutaminase antibody (anti-tTG) and anti-reticulin antibody (ARA) occur in the serum and gastrointestinal secretions, and the rash is gluten sensitive. The importance of these factors and how they interact to produce skin lesions remains unknown, though recently antibodies directed at epidermal transglutaminase (TG3) have been identified in patients with DH and this may be the dominant autoantigen in the disorder.

An early hypothesis proposed that gluten–anti-gluten immune complexes were central in the pathogenesis of DH and, by binding to reticulin in the skin, produced the lesions. Gluten, however, has never been found in skin lesions, though it may be present in a form that is difficult to detect. IgA is present in uninvolved skin, and is still present when the rash goes into remission, either spontaneously or following treatment. It is difficult to quantify IgA in the skin and, even on a strict gluten-free diet (GFD), it can take several years for this to clear from the skin.

Clinical features

Rash. The earliest abnormality consists of a small erythematous macule, 2–3 mm in diameter, which rapidly develops into an urticarial papule. Small vesicles appear, which may coalesce; if scratched, they may rupture, dry and form scabs. The vesicles are tense shiny and filled with clear fluid, which clouds as the lesion progresses. Pustules are rare. Blisters take 7–10 days to involute and, at any one time, all stages of development will be present.

The predominant symptoms are intense itching and burning. Rupture of the blisters by scratching leads to rapid relief of symptoms and only evidence of excoriation may be seen at presentation. Healing is often complete, but areas of pigmentation and occasionally scars may remain. The rash has a characteristic symmetrical distribution and can be found on any part of the body except the soles of the feet. The elbows and

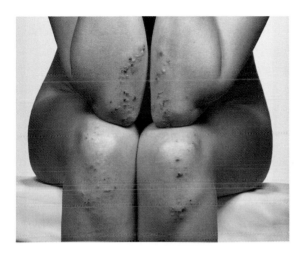

Figure 7.1 Blisters on the elbows and knees of a patient with dermatitis herpetiformis. Reproduced courtesy of T Reunala, Tampere, Finland.

upper forearms are affected in over 90% of patients (Figure 7.1). Other sites commonly involved are the buttocks, knees, shoulders, sacrum, face, scalp, neck and trunk. Oral lesions are found in 5% of cases. The rash may be widespread, but can be limited to one or two sites. Local trauma caused by, for example, belts, braces and straps, may precipitate lesions and, following inadequate drug treatment, the rash tends to reappear at the same sites.

Once the rash appears, it is a continuous problem in most patients, but it can run an intermittent course in 10% of cases. Lesions may be worse premenstrually, though pregnancy has a variable effect. DH tends to be less severe in the elderly and may be more likely to remit spontaneously. For those taking a normal diet, the spontaneous remission rate is around 10%, but the diagnosis in these atypical patients should be reviewed.

Associated enteropathy. Over 90% of patients with DH have no gastrointestinal symptoms. This may be because the mucosal abnormalities extend only a short distance into the small intestine leaving sufficient normal bowel to compensate. A few patients do, however, complain of diarrhea or abdominal bloating, but severe symptoms are rare.

Villous atrophy in the upper small-intestinal mucosa is found in 65–75% of patients with DH. Lesions are often patchy, and taking

85

multiple biopsies using a fiber-optic endoscope increases the likelihood of detecting abnormalities. Even in patients with apparently normal biopsies, subtle changes in the mucosa such as raised numbers of intraepithelial lymphocytes (IELs) and γ/δ T cells in the epithelium, alterations in intestinal humoral immunity and the production of villous atrophy with gluten challenge, indicate gluten sensitivity.

Associated endocrine and connective tissue disorders. DH is associated with endocrine or connective tissue disorders in about 5% of patients, and these problems usually develop prior to the diagnosis of DH. The most common endocrine problems are autoimmune thyroid disease and type 1 diabetes mellitus; the connective tissue disorders include Sjögren's syndrome, lupus erythematosus, rheumatoid arthritis and scleroderma. It is important that these associated conditions are not overlooked at diagnosis of DH or during follow up.

Malignancy. Lymphoma or other types of malignancy may complicate DH and occur before, coincidentally with or after the diagnosis of DH is established.

Prognosis. The prognosis is good unless lymphoma develops, but this is unusual. It should be possible to control the rash with drugs and a GFD, though relapses may occur for no apparent reason from time to time.

Investigations

Histological findings in the skin are non-specific and take the form of papillary microabscesses and subepidermal blisters with a neutrophil infiltration. A 4-mm punch biopsy should be taken and snap frozen in liquid nitrogen for immunofluorescence studies, which can detect IgA deposits in the skin.

IgA deposits in skin. The diagnosis of DH rests on the demonstration of IgA in uninvolved skin. The most common site is in the dermal papillae, where IgA is detected as granular or fibrillar deposits (Figure 7.2). IgA may also be laid down in a linear granular fashion along the line of the basement membrane. It is important that this

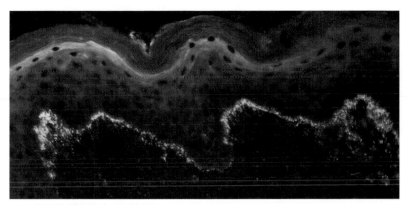

Figure 7.2 Immunofluorescence biopsy showing granular IgA deposits in the upper papillary dermis in a patient with dermatitis herpetiformis. Reproduced courtesy of T Reunala, Tampere, Finland.

pattern is differentiated from homogeneous linear IgA deposition found in linear IgA disease (LAD), which is not gluten dependent. It has been claimed that if multiple sections of skin of one or two biopsies are carefully examined by a skilled observer, all patients with DH will show IgA deposits. The corollary of this is that the diagnosis of DH should not be accepted in the absence of these abnormalities.

Small-bowel biopsy. A biopsy of the upper small bowel is required in all patients. These are usually obtained from the duodenum using standard fiber-optic endoscopes, which allow several specimens to be taken. If the biopsy appears to be normal or near normal by routine histology, more sophisticated tests will indicate subtle changes indicating gluten sensitivity as outlined above.

Tests of malabsorption. Although patients may not have overt evidence of malabsorption, hemoglobin, ferritin, folate and vitamin B_{12} concentrations should be measured because deficiencies may exist. Low serum calcium and elevated alkaline phosphatase will indicate osteomalacia.

Imaging is required only if sinister symptoms, such as those suggestive of small-bowel lymphoma, are present.

Differential diagnosis

While DH can be easily recognized in most cases because of its characteristic presentation, appearance and distribution, other disorders have to be considered in less typical cases. Difficulties arise when lesions are sparse and scratching has left only excoriations and scabs. In addition, rashes in some other conditions may appear clinically similar to DH and respond to sulfones. Disorders that have to be differentiated include eczema, LAD, pemphigoid and pemphigus.

Eczema. The distribution of eczema differs from that of DH and is not confined to extensor surfaces. The lesions respond to topical and systemic steroids, and tests for immunofluorescence are negative. In some patients, dapsone will reduce the itch, which may cause diagnostic confusion.

Linear IgA disease. The blisters in LAD are similar to those seen in DH, but are not confined to extensor surfaces. A skin biopsy will show IgA deposited characteristically in a linear fashion along the dermato–epidermal junction. LAD of childhood also shows this staining pattern and the rash responds to dapsone.

Pemphigoid occurs in an older population and the tense blisters vary in size from a few millimeters to a few centimeters. The groin, axillae, flexures of the limbs and lower abdomen are most commonly involved. IgG is found at the dermato–epidermal junction. The disorder responds to steroids and, after treatment for 2–3 years, many patients remain in remission.

Pemphigus is characterized by thin-walled blisters, which are present in the mouth in 50% of cases. The intraepithelial blisters rupture easily to leave eroded areas prone to secondary infection. If lesions are extensive, fluid loss can lead to severe metabolic changes and death. Intercellular IgG is present in the skin. Steroids have improved the prognosis, but may contribute to mortality because of side effects.

Treatment

The rash of DH responds rapidly to drug treatment, which is required by almost all patients because of severe irritation. A GFD should be advised and enables most patients ultimately to stop or reduce the drug dose. Supplements should be given to patients with nutritional deficiencies (e.g. iron, folate).

Drug treatments. The two drugs commonly used to control the rash are dapsone and sulfapyridine. Remission is induced within 24–48 hours and the rash clears within a week. These agents are so effective that if treatment fails the diagnosis should be reviewed. Lesions return rapidly if the drugs are withdrawn before a GFD has had time to act.

Dapsone is the most widely used agent. Initially, it should be given in a dose of 100 mg, which is effective in most patients. Larger doses may be used, but are seldom required. It is not usually possible to reduce the dose until the patient has been on a GFD for about 6 months. Side effects include anorexia, nausea, vomiting, insomnia, headache, neuropathy and hypoalbuminemia. Hemolysis is common, as evidenced by a macrocytosis; methemoglobinemia is also common. These side effects are rarely of clinical importance but an indication to change to another agent.

Sulfapyridine may be used instead of, or in combination with, dapsone.

Gluten-free diet. All patients should be offered a GFD, even when the small-intestinal mucosa appears normal, because the rash of DH is gluten sensitive. They should be interviewed by a dietitian and advised to adhere strictly to the diet. Patients may be reluctant to start or continue with a GFD, because only a few have gastrointestinal symptoms, which are usually mild. Following a GFD and with the benefit of hindsight, however, many patients do experience more energy and a greater sense of wellbeing. If it is carefully explained that this course of action may have a beneficial effect on their skin and avoid the necessity for long-term medication, patients are much more likely to comply. Other benefits of a GFD include a reduction in the risk of malignant and non-malignant complications.

Whether patients can stop medication depends on their adherence to, and time on, a GFD. Of those patients who adhere strictly to a GFD, over 90% will be able to discontinue medication after 2 years. Fewer than 50% of those who continue to ingest some gluten are able to stop drug treatment, and the time to achieve this is 4–6 years. Those who elect to take a normal diet will require medication to suppress the rash unless they go into spontaneous remission.

Key points – dermatitis herpetiformis

- Dermatitis herpetiformis (DH) is a blistering itchy rash that has a characteristic symmetrical distribution and is found mainly on the extensor surfaces of the elbows and knees.
- DH is closely linked to celiac disease.
- Only a minority, about 10%, of patients have gastrointestinal symptoms and these are usually mild.
- The diagnosis rests on finding IgA deposits by immunofluorescence in skin uninvolved by the rash.
- The rash is gluten sensitive and all patients should adhere to a strict gluten-free diet (GFD).
- Dapsone is a very effective treatment and can be stopped after about 2 years in 90% of those who adhere to a strict GFD.

Key references

Fry L. Dermatitis herpetiformis. *Baillière's Clin Gastroenterol* 1995;9:371–93.

Garioch JJ, Lewis HM, Sargent SA et al. 25 years' experience of a gluten-free diet in the treatment of dermatitis herpetiformis. *Br J Dermatol* 1994;131:541–5.

Hull CM, Liddle M, Hansen N et al. Elevation of IgA anti-epidermal transglutaminase antibodies in dermatitis herpetiformis. *Br J Dermatol* 2008;159:120–4.

Reunala T, Collin P. Diseases associated with dermatitis herpetiformis. *Br J Dermatol* 1997;136:315–18.

Patients with celiac disease, particularly those who are undiagnosed or do not adhere to a strict gluten-free diet (GFD), are prone to develop complications. Malignant complications are the most serious and should be suspected when expected responses to a GFD are not achieved or sustained. Lymphoma and other malignant tumors, particularly carcinoma of the esophagus and jejunum, are associated with celiac disease.

Etiology

The etiology of malignant complications is unknown, but local and general mechanisms have to be considered (Table 8.1).

Prevalence

The prevalence of malignant complications has been difficult to ascertain for several reasons.

- The prevalence of celiac disease in the population is unknown because many patients who do not have symptoms or have only mild complaints may never be diagnosed.

TABLE 8.1

Mechanisms that may underlie the development of malignancy

- The mucosal lesion is premalignant
- Carcinogens may penetrate the abnormally permeable mucosa
- The mucosa may be deficient in carcinogen-detoxifying enzymes
- Abnormalities in the immune system may predispose to tumor formation
- Immune disturbances may allow oncogenic viruses to replicate
- The HLA status may predispose to malignancy

HLA, human leukocyte antigen.

- If autopsies are not performed, the presence of malignancy will be underestimated.
- Patients with lymphoma or other malignancy may have celiac disease that remains undiagnosed.
- Data reported from referral centers are unlikely to reflect the fate of celiac patients in the general population.
- The wider use of a GFD is altering the risk of developing lymphoma.
- Some celiac populations may be at greater risk than others.

Recent studies have demonstrated that the malignant risk is lower than previously thought.

A study from Italy of patients with newly diagnosed non-Hodgkin lymphoma (NHL) and population controls that used anti-endomysial antibody (AEA) as the screening test for celiac disease found the increased risk of NHL of any primary site was 3.1, for NHL in the gut 16.9 and for T-cell NHL 19.2.

A large population-based investigation from Sweden found an overall risk of cancer in celiac disease of 1.3 using standardized incidence ratios. The increased risk for NHL was a modest 6.3. Of interest, and confirmed in other studies, the risk of breast cancer was reduced – this finding is unexplained.

Under the auspices of the British Society of Gastroenterology, a postal survey was undertaken of small-bowel malignancy in the UK during 1998–2000. Over this period, 107 lymphomas and 175 adenocarcinomas were reported, of which 42 (39%) and 23 (13%), respectively, were associated with celiac disease. Thus, in the whole celiac population of the UK only about 20 small-bowel lymphomas and 12 small-bowel adenocarcinomas will occur each year.

An investigation employing the UK general practice research database found that patients with celiac disease had only a modestly increased risk of malignancy and mortality compared with the general population. The hazard ratio for any malignancy was 1.29, for lymphoproliferative disease 4.80 and for mortality 1.31. A reduction in breast cancer was also confirmed.

A study from a single center in Southern Derbyshire, England, of patients with celiac disease followed for 24 years found a five-times greater rate of NHL and a 40-times greater rate of small-bowel lymphoma than in the general population. Only 3 patients with enteropathy-associated T-cell lymphoma, 2 with esophageal and 2 with small-bowel adenocarcinoma were encountered.

A European multicenter investigation involving ten countries found an odds ratio for developing NHL of 2.6. This increased risk was only found in those with clinically diagnosed celiac disease and not in those with silent celiac disease detected by screening.

The evidence indicates that the absolute numbers of malignancies complicating celiac disease are small, so that patients can be reassured that there is a very low chance that cancer will develop. There is a decreasing risk of malignant lymphoma with time, which may reflect the beneficial effects of strict adherence to a GFD, which is known to have a protective influence. The decreasing risk over time may also extend to buccal, esophageal and small-intestinal carcinoma. Patients are extremely unlikely to develop a lymphoma if they survive 3–5 years following the diagnosis of celiac disease and maintain a strict GFD. Children do not appear to be at risk of developing lymphoma and those with dermatitis herpetiformis have only a small risk.

Lymphoma

Lymphoma is of T-cell origin and is referred to as enteropathy-associated T-cell lymphoma (EATL) (see *Fast Facts: Lymphoma*). This type of lymphoma can occur in the absence of enteropathy, suggesting that EATL is a clinical rather than pathological entity. A monoclonal antibody called HML-1, developed against intraepithelial lymphocytes (IELs), also stains these lymphoma cells. In celiac disease, there is an expansion of the $CD3^+$, $CD7^+$, $CD4^-$ and $CD8^-$ IEL population and the phenotype of EATL suggests an origin from these double-negative cells.

Clinical presentation. Lymphoma in patients with celiac disease presents in one of two ways.

The diagnosis of celiac disease clearly precedes the onset of symptoms attributed to malignancy. These patients have responded to a GFD then deteriorate because of the onset of lymphoma.

Celiac disease and lymphoma present together, or within a short interval of time. Whether these patients have long-standing untreated

93

celiac disease has been the subject of controversy. However, evidence indicates that the development of lymphoma is the event that brings celiac disease to attention. When compared with uncomplicated patients with celiac disease, this group has a similar HLA profile, similar changes in intraepithelial subsets and a similar incidence of hyposplenism. Furthermore, the presence of the HLA class II alleles associated with celiac disease, *DQA1*0501;DQB1*0201*, and immunohistochemical studies of EATL also support this view.

Weight loss, lethargy, diarrhea, abdominal pain, muscle weakness, finger-clubbing, pyrexia and lymphadenopathy are symptoms that point to the diagnosis of lymphoma. In most patients the illness is insidious, but presentation can be acute with intestinal perforation, obstruction or bleeding from the tumor (Figures 8.1 and 8.2).

Diagnosis. The diagnosis of lymphoma can be difficult and delayed because the presenting features are often non-specific and similar to those encountered in celiac disease at diagnosis or in relapse. In about one-third of cases, the diagnosis is made only at autopsy.

Hematology/biochemistry. Many hematologic and biochemical abnormalities occur in celiac patients with lymphoma, but no pattern that allows early diagnosis has been found. A progressive rise in serum immunoglobulin A is sometimes seen, but this may also occur in celiac disease without malignancy. Serum lysozyme increases, but this is not a reliable indicator of lymphoma. Lower plasma cell and higher

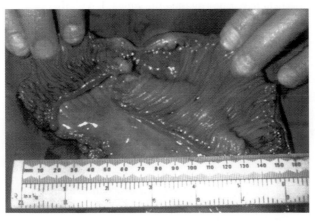

Figure 8.1
Obstructing lymphoma in the jejunum.

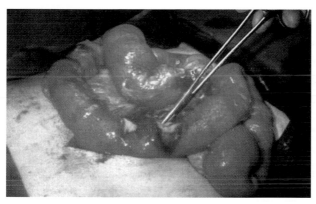

Figure 8.2
Multifocal enteropathy-associated T-cell lymphoma with perforation.

lymphocyte counts in the lamina propria and lower lymphocyte counts in the epithelium have been reported in small-bowel biopsies from patients who eventually develop lymphoma compared with those who do not. Hypoplastic crypts and histiocytic aggregates have also been reported. Unfortunately, these observations are not helpful in individual patients.

Imaging. Small-bowel radiography employing either a barium meal and follow through or by delivering barium directly in to the small bowel (enteroclysis) is essential if lymphoma is suspected and will reveal multiple irregular narrowed segments characteristic of small-bowel involvement (Figure 8.3). Lesions may not, however, be evident on radiography and only a malabsorption pattern seen.

Computed tomography (CT) with intravenous and oral contrast can also be used. In addition to intraluminal pathology, CT will also

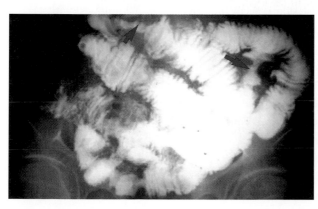

Figure 8.3
Barium study showing two lymphomatous strictures (arrowed) in the small bowel.

95

provide information on, for example, the thickness of the bowel wall, lymph nodes and the size of the spleen, some or all of which may be abnormal in the presence of lymphoma.

Alternatively, exposure of patients to radiation can be avoided by a magnetic resonance imaging (MRI) contrast study of the small bowel, which will also give similar intra- and extraluminal information if lymphoma is present. Positron emission tomography (PET) may help to identify malignant tissue and the response to treatment.

Upper gastrointestinal endoscopy, which is now the preferred method for diagnosing celiac disease, also allows inspection of the esophagus, stomach and proximal duodenum, but more distal bowel needs to be visualized. Push or double-balloon endoscopy allows this, but respiratory distress, aspiration pneumonia and intestinal perforation are uncommon complications. These techniques allow direct inspection of the bowel; biopsies can be taken to confirm malignancy or jejunoileitis, which is also a cause for deterioration in celiac disease and may be associated with lymphoma.

Video capsule endoscopy allows the whole of the small bowel to be inspected but not biopsied. The presence of strictures limits this technique, because the capsule can become trapped. Strictures must, therefore, be excluded by methods referred to above before a capsule is introduced into the small bowel.

Investigation. A strategy to investigate for lymphoma would be first to visualize the small bowel with MRI, which will also give extraluminal information. If a lesion is seen, the MRI should be followed with enteroscopy so that biopsies of suspicious areas can be obtained. Enlarged lymph nodes or other masses should be biopsied under ultrasound control. Alternatively, tissue can be obtained at laparoscopy. If MRI does not show focal lesions but the suspicion of lymphoma remains, video capsule endoscopy can be carried out, followed by enteroscopy if lesions are seen. Laparotomy may be necessary when lymphoma is suspected, but a firm diagnosis cannot be made. This can be a difficult decision in an ill patient as surgery may contribute to mortality. On the other hand, it is sometimes possible to perform a curative operation for a localized lesion.

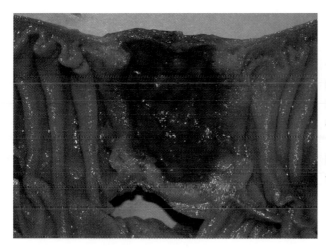

Figure 8.4
Enteropathy-
associated
T-cell
lymphoma in
the jejunum.

Pathology. In patients with celiac disease, 80% of lymphomas are located in the duodenum or jejunum compared with 45% in those without celiac disease. They may also be found in the ileum and lymph nodes and, less commonly, in the stomach and colon. They occur as solitary or multiple circumferential ulcerating lesions, mucosal plaques or nodules (Figure 8.4). Stenoses of the bowel may occur. The histological appearance varies, but the tumors are of high grade and large cell type (Figure 8.5). The mucosa of the adjacent bowel is flat.

Carcinoma

As for lymphoma, the development of carcinoma may bring a patient with celiac disease to diagnosis or provoke symptoms in a patient whose condition was previously well controlled on a GFD.

Carcinoma of the esophagus usually presents with dysphagia, anemia or bleeding and can be diagnosed by biopsy at endoscopy.

Carcinoma of the jejunum. The lesions in patients with celiac disease are more commonly found in the proximal bowel (95%) with equal distribution between the duodenum and jejunum, compared with the distribution in patients without celiac disease (70%) (Figure 8.6). Anemia is the most common presenting feature and is often associated with either overt or occult gastrointestinal blood loss. Weight loss,

97

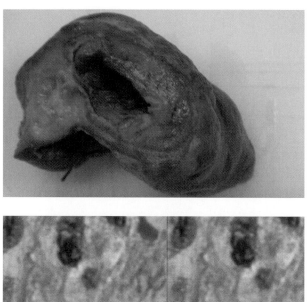

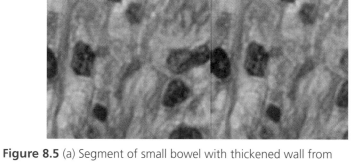

Figure 8.5 (a) Segment of small bowel with thickened wall from enteropathy-associated T-cell lymphoma. (b) Histology revealed large irregular pleomorphic lymphoid cells. Markers confirmed enteropathy-associated T-cell lymphoma. Enteropathy was evident in adjacent mucosa.

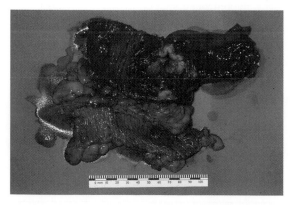

Figure 8.6
Adenocarcinoma of the jejunum complicating celiac disease. A small segment of adherent colon was also resected.

abdominal pain and intestinal obstruction are other prominent complaints. If the tumor is in the proximal duodenum, it may be visualized at endoscopy. Barium studies will usually detect lesions further down the intestine or show evidence of obstruction; this area can then be inspected and biopsied at enteroscopy.

Other carcinomas. There is evidence for an increase in the incidence of oropharyngeal and primary liver cancer and also of cancer of the right and ascending colon and some endocrine tumors. Several studies indicate a reduction in breast cancer, which remains unexplained, though it could be related to lower bodyweight of celiac patients and their lower rates of smoking.

Risk of malignancy in other groups

Dermatitis herpetiformis. Whether patients with dermatitis herpetiformis have an increased risk of developing lymphoma is disputed. One study indicates no risk and another a twofold increase in risk. It is likely that there is an increased risk but that this is smaller than occurs in celiac disease. There appears to be no increased risk of developing carcinoma of the gastrointestinal tract.

Relatives of patients with celiac disease. No increase in risk of lymphoma has been observed, but a higher risk of esophageal cancer has been found.

Refractory celiac disease is defined as persisting villous atrophy, usually with symptoms of severe malabsorption, in those who have maintained a strict GFD for at least 1 year and where other specific causes have been excluded. Refractory celiac disease can be divided into types 1 and 2, which account for 25% and 75% of the whole group, respectively. Type 1 has a normal intraepithelial cell population and carries a good prognosis. Treatment with steroids and azathioprine are effective and the 5-year survival is over 95%. Type 2 has an aberrant clonal intraepithelial cell population. The cells carry intracytoplasmic but not surface CD3, usually lack CD8 and have clonal rearrangements of the T-cell receptor (TCR)-γ gene. A simple diagnostic method using anti-

CD3 and anti-CD8 antibodies on paraffin sections has been described; routine histopathology laboratories should be able to develop this to distinguish active celiac disease resulting from poor adherence to a GFD from type 2 refractory celiac disease.

Type 2 refractory disease carries a poor prognosis, and 50–60% of patients develop a lymphoma within 5 years. Treatments are of very limited value and have included azathioprine, ciclosporin, cladribine and autologous stem-cell transplantation. Effective treatments are urgently required because elimination of the aberrant neoplastic cells would halt the progression to overt lymphoma. EATL can arise either directly from the aberrant intraepithelial lymphocytes or after passing through a stage of refractory sprue, which may manifest as chronic ulcerative jejunoileitis. In this condition ulcers are found mainly in the jejunum and ileum (see pages 80–1; Figure 8.7). It can be difficult to differentiate from bowel lymphoma clinically and radiologically. In addition, both disorders may occur together in the same patient and sometimes ulceration will be diagnosed before lymphoma becomes apparent.

Treatment and prognosis

Surgery, radiotherapy and chemotherapy may be used in suitable cases depending on the site of lesions and staging. If tumors are confined to the gastrointestinal tract, resection of the affected segment (or segments) may result in cure. In most patients, lymphoma is widespread at diagnosis and the outlook is poor. Survival rates at 1 year and at 5 years in one series were 31% and 11%, respectively, and 39% and 20% in another. In a national British survey of lymphoma in celiac disease, survival at 30 months was only 13%.

Effect of gluten-free diet

Because of the difficulties in making an early diagnosis of lymphoma and the poor prognosis, attention has turned to prevention and the role that a GFD might play. A GFD restores the structure and function of the small bowel towards normal and might, therefore, reduce the malignant potential.

A study investigating the effect of a GFD on the risk of malignancy was carried out in Birmingham, UK. Of the 210 patients, 108 followed

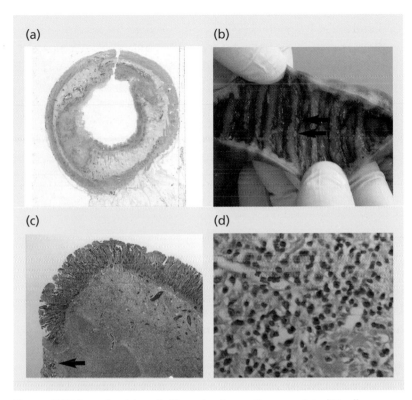

Figure 8.7 Ulcerative jejunoileitis and enteropathy-associated T-cell lymphoma (EATL). (a) Cross section of resected jejunum showing mucosa covering only a quarter of the bowel luminal surface. (b) Luminal surface of jejunum showing extensive mucosal ulceration with only small islands of intact mucosa surviving (arrowed). (c) Section of jejunum showing crypt hyperplasia and villous atrophy but with an area of ulceration on the left. Underneath is a dense lymphoid infiltrate. (d) An apparently bland submucosal infiltrate which required molecular markers to establish EATL.

a strict GFD, while the remainder had a normal or reduced-gluten diet. In the group that had taken a strict GFD for 5 or more consecutive years, the overall risk of malignancy was not significantly increased compared with that of the general population. For those ingesting gluten, however, the risk was significantly increased. Excess morbidity was also calculated and was clearly related to the amount of gluten ingested (Table 8.2).

TABLE 8.2

Effect of diet on morbidity from cancer of the mouth, pharynx and esophagus, and lymphoma in patients with celiac disease

Diet	Number of patients	Morbidity rate	
		Observed	Expected
Normal	46	7	0.19
Reduced gluten	56	5	0.12
Strict gluten-free	108	3	0.46

*Excess morbidity rate = observed – expected/ person years at risk × 10^3.
Trend for excess morbidity rate over diet group: $\chi_1^2 = 9.9$; $p < 0.01$.

Study of lymphoma in dermatitis herpetiformis has also shown a GFD to be protective. These results are supported by other studies and indicate that a GFD does reduce the malignant risk and is a further reason to advise all patients to adhere to a strict diet for life.

Approach to patients

Patients are becoming increasingly aware of the link between celiac disease and malignancy, and would like further information. This is a very sensitive area and a thoughtful approach is required so that patients do not become unduly alarmed. It is now possible to adopt an encouraging and positive attitude by explaining to patients that malignant complications only rarely occur and an effective way to avoid them is by adhering to a strict GFD for life.

Observed/expected	p value	Excess morbidity rate*
36.8	< 0.001	10.7
41.7	< 0.001	5.0
6.5	< 0.05	1.2

Key points – malignant complications

- Patients with celiac disease who do not respond to a strict gluten-free diet (GFD) or who relapse on diet may have developed a serious complication.
- Celiac disease is associated with lymphoma and other forms of cancer, particularly of the esophagus and small intestine. Enteropathy-associated T-cell lymphoma is a rare form of high-grade non-Hodgkin lymphoma of the upper small intestine that is specifically associated with celiac disease.
- The frequency of these complications is lower than previously thought and the absolute number of cancers arising is small, so patients can be reassured that their chance of developing malignancy is very low. Following a strict GFD reduces the lymphoma risk.
- Type 2 refractory celiac disease is a forerunner of overt lymphoma and new treatments to eliminate the aberrant cells are urgently needed.

Key references

Askling J, Linet M, Gridley G et al. Cancer incidence in a population-based cohort of individuals hospitalized with celiac disease or dermatitis herpetiformis. *Gastroenterology* 2002;123: 1428–35.

Card TR, West J, Holmes GKT. Risk of malignancy in diagnosed coeliac disease: a 24-year prospective, population-based, cohort study. *Aliment Pharmacol Ther* 2004;20:769–75.

Catassi C, Bearzi I, Holmes GKT. Association of celiac disease and intestinal lymphomas and other cancers. *Gastroenterology* 2005; 128(4 Suppl 1):S79–86.

Catassi C, Fabiani E, Corrao G et al. Risk of non-Hodgkin lymphoma in celiac disease. *JAMA* 2002;287: 1413–19.

Cellier C, Delabesse E, Helmer C et al. Refractory sprue, coeliac disease, and enteropathy-associated T-cell lymphoma. *Lancet* 2000;356: 203–8.

Di Sabatino A, Rosado MM, Cazzola P et al. Splenic hypofunction and the spectrum of autoimmune and malignant complications in celiac disease. *Clin Gastroenterol Hepatol* 2006;4:179–86.

Hatton C, Collins G, Sweetenham J. *Fast Facts: Lymphoma*. Oxford: Health Press, 2008.

Holmes GKT, Prior P, Lane MR et al. Malignancy in coeliac disease – effect of a gluten free diet. *Gut* 1989;30: 333–8.

Howdle PD, Jalal PK, Holmes GKT, Houlston RS. Primary small-bowel malignancy in the UK and its association with coeliac disease. *QJM* 2003;96:345–53.

Mearin ML, Catassi C, Brousse N et al. European multi-centre study on coeliac disease and non-Hodgkin lymphoma. *Eur J Gastroenterol Hepatol* 2006;18;187–94.

Patey-Mariaud de Serre N, Cellier C, Jabri B et al. Distinction between coeliac disease and refractory sprue: a simple immunohistochemical method. *Histopathology* 2000;37:70–7.

West J, Logan RFA, Smith CJ et al. Malignancy and mortality in people with coeliac disease: population based cohort study. *BMJ* 2004; 329:716–19.

Management

The treatment of celiac disease is based on the lifelong exclusion of gluten-containing cereals from the diet. In many areas of the world, including Europe, North America, Australasia and North Africa, gluten-rich products such as bread and pasta are part of the staple diet. Gluten-containing foods make a substantial contribution to daily energy intake and are enjoyable to eat. The changes needed to begin and maintain a gluten-free diet (GFD) are substantial and have a major impact on daily life. Thus, starting the diet is a critical step that should be handled sympathetically by experienced doctors and dietitians. The rationale for and the benefits of the diet require careful explanation, placing emphasis on the wide range of foods that can be eaten rather than just on those that have to be excluded.

The gluten-free diet

Wheat, barley and rye proteins are completely excluded in the GFD. Kamut, Emkorn and Spelt are varieties of wheat that must also be excluded. Rice, maize and buckwheat do not contain gluten and can be eaten. Potato, chestnut, tapioca, sorghum, millet, teff, quinoa and amaranth are other safe starchy foods. In the past, oats were considered to be toxic to individuals with celiac disease. Many recent studies, however, have shown that the ingestion of uncontaminated oats is not only safe but can also improve the quality of the diet in the majority of patients with either celiac disease or dermatitis herpetiformis. The abdominal discomfort reported by some patients after ingesting oats is merely related to increased intake of dietary fiber. Oats contribute much-valued variety, taste, satiety, dietary fiber and other essential nutrients to the celiac diet. Other natural foods such as vegetables, salads, pulses, fruits, nuts, meat, fish, poultry, cheese, eggs and milk can be consumed in the GFD without limitation. A wide range of attractive and palatable gluten-free products that guarantee the absence of gluten are specifically manufactured for celiac patients and may be labeled by an internationally recognized mark, the crossed ear of wheat.

Nutritional adequacy. Gluten is a protein with limited nutritional value that can be substituted by other dietary proteins. The intake of some nutrients tends to be lower than normal with the GFD, particularly fiber, iron, calcium and folate, and these should be carefully monitored. Limiting the intake of gluten-free snacks rich in simple sugars and fat is also prudent to avoid excessive weight gain and/or blood lipid abnormalities.

Hidden gluten. Many commercial products, ready meals and convenience foods are made with wheat flour, gluten-containing wheat proteins or gluten-containing starches, which are added as a filler, stabilizing agent or processing aid. These include sausages, fish fingers, cheese spreads, soups, sauces, mixed seasonings, mincemeat for mince pies, and some medications and vitamin preparations. Although gluten-free beers have recently appeared on the market, most real ales, beers, lagers and stout should be avoided, but spirits, wines, liqueurs and ciders are allowed. Whisky and malt whisky are allowed.

National celiac societies in many countries publish handbooks that list the gluten-free products available. Celiac societies will have ascertained from food manufacturers which products are safe and these are included in the food lists. These handbooks are regularly updated and are essential for celiac patients to have in their possession. It is important to remember that food lists are only applicable for use in the country in which they were compiled. Similar foods with well-known brand names may be made under franchise in different countries to slightly different recipes; they may look and taste the same, but be gluten free in one country and not in others.

Food labeling is an important issue for celiac patients who need to exclude gluten-containing ingredients from their diet. Food labeling directives have been improved by the Codex Alimentarius, a joint Commission of the Food and Agriculture Organization of the United Nations and the World Health Organization, representing 98% of the world's countries. According to the current Codex regulations, foods and ingredients that are known to cause hypersensitive reactions, including gluten-containing cereals such as wheat, barley and rye, must always be declared on the label without exception if they are part of a compound ingredient or have been added for technological reasons or processing purposes. The following non-toxic ingredients are, however, exempt from compulsory labels:

- wheat-based glucose syrups and maltodextrins
- barley-based glucose syrups and cereals used in distillates for spirits.

In 2003 the Codex directive was adopted by the European Parliament and consequently brought into force in the member states. In the USA, the Food Allergen Labeling and Consumer Protection Act was implemented in 2004. These directives have simplified label reading by identifying those foods that contain hidden wheat gluten.

Gluten contamination. Although zero gluten intake is the ideal treatment for celiac disease, in the real world a degree of gluten contamination is unavoidable. Not only may gluten be hidden in many commercial foods but grains that are naturally gluten free may become cross-contaminated with wheat, particularly during milling, storage and other manipulations. Wheat starch is a purified compound that can contain traces of residual gluten. This wheat derivate has been used in the UK and other Northern European countries as an ingredient for gluten-free foods for many years.

Simple immunoenzymatic methods, such as the R5 enzyme-linked immunosorbent assay (ELISA), are available for measuring the level of gluten contamination in food. However, certain analytical difficulties still need to be resolved (e.g. the analysis of hydrolyzed products or the glutenin component in wheat).

Although the potential toxicity of small amounts of gluten is still disputed, recent studies have had interesting results. The lowest amount of daily gluten that induces damage to the small-intestinal mucosa (gluten threshold) on a long-term basis is 10–50 mg per day (Figure 9.1). There is wide interpatient variability in the sensitivity to trace amounts of gluten both at the clinical and histological level, and occasionally a patient may react to even a few mg of daily gluten. The intake of small amounts of gluten taken with gluten-free food depends on the amount of wheat substitutes that are consumed on a daily basis, which mostly varies between 100 and 500 g per day in different

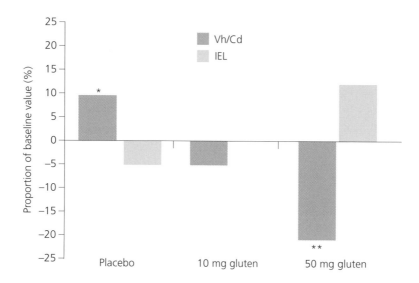

Figure 9.1 Effects of a 3-month gluten 'micro' challenge on morphometric indices of the small-intestinal mucosa in celiac patients. After the micro challenge, patients challenged with the placebo showed an increase of the villus height:crypt depth (Vh/Cd) ratio that was not seen in those receiving either 10 or 50 mg of daily gluten. Patients challenged with 50 mg of daily gluten showed a significant deterioration of the Vh/Cd compared with the placebo group. IEL, intraepithelial lymphocytes. *Significantly improved; **significantly different from placebo. Data from Catassi et al., 2007.

countries. This information has been used to define the maximum amount of gluten that can be allowed in foods that are suitable for patients with celiac disease (Figure 9.2). The new Codex standard has two categories: products containing less than 20 parts per million (ppm) (1 ppm = 1 mg/kg) of gluten will be labeled as 'gluten free', while products containing between 20 and 100 ppm of gluten will be labeled as 'very low gluten'. These measures will become law in January 2012.

Compliance with the gluten-free diet

Studies have shown that between 45% and 94% of patients adhere to a strict GFD. This wide variation reflects, to some extent, whether the study population was made up of children or adults, the proportion

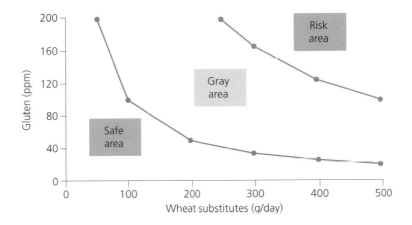

Figure 9.2 Relationship between the level of gluten contamination (expressed in parts per million [ppm]) in nominally gluten-free products and the amount of wheat substitutes (e.g. bread and pasta) eaten every day. The risky ingestion of 50 mg of daily gluten can be reached in individuals eating a large amount of wheat substitutes (500 g/day) containing 100 ppm of gluten. The toxicity of 10–50 mg per day of gluten remains a gray area that requires further investigation.

with few or no symptoms, and the closeness of follow up. Strict dietary compliance is a problem for a number of reasons (Table 9.1).

Risk associated with ingesting small amounts of gluten

Quite apart from non-compliance, gluten may be present in a diet apparently free from gluten for the reasons outlined previously. Patients often ask whether eating small amounts of gluten regularly or occasionally will be harmful. The best advice is that they should adhere strictly to the diet, but it has to be conceded that the risks associated with the protracted ingestion of very small amounts of gluten are still unclear. Although most patients will not experience any clinical symptoms if they eat small amounts of gluten, it has been shown that intestinal mucosal architecture may deteriorate with an increasing intraepithelial lymphocyte (IEL) count, which is the most sensitive index to detect abnormalities (see Figure 9.1).

TABLE 9.1

Possible reasons for poor adherence to a gluten-free diet

- Imposes restrictions on everyday lifestyle
- Particularly difficult to maintain when traveling, eating out, dining with friends and on holiday
- Adolescents:
  - peer pressure and a sense of not wanting to be different from their friends
  - gluten can be ingested without producing symptoms in this age group
- Silent celiac disease (i.e. a flat biopsy but no symptoms): little incentive to adhere strictly to the diet because patients regard themselves as well
- Expense of gluten-free foods

Psychosocial burden

Although it is indisputable that the GFD is one of the most effective and safe treatments available in medicine, the emotional and social implications of lifelong living without gluten should not be underestimated. The lifestyle changes required and the additional financial burden imposed by a GFD, particularly in countries where no economic support is provided by the healthcare system (e.g. the USA), can have a negative impact. Although patients who have long been searching for a cause to explain their ill health are relieved by the diagnosis of celiac disease, quality of life, self-perceived health and mental health tend to decline over time. These effects are stronger among women than men and depression is frequently encountered in treated adults.

Emotions, relationships and the management of daily life are the main categories of concern experienced by adolescents and adults with celiac disease. Specific feelings reported in relation to the disease include a sense of isolation, shame, fear of ingesting gluten and worries about being a burden on others. Frequent dilemmas associated with interpersonal relationships are unwanted visibility, neglect, being forgotten, disclosure avoidance and risk-taking with the diet. Dilemmas related to the management of daily life revolve around restricted product choice and the effort involved in preparing meals.

Sympathetic support, education and attention to changing nutritional needs are critical factors in the adaptation of patients to the new diet and lifestyle. Ideally, a team approach – with the team comprising the patient, physician, dietitian and local support group – should be employed when educating the newly diagnosed patient about a GFD. In selected cases (e.g. vulnerable adolescents), professional psychological support may be required.

Other treatments

While virtually all children respond well to a GFD, 10–15% of adult patients do not and additional measures have to be employed. Initially, the following interventions can be tried; these will settle the symptoms of some patients completely.

Restriction of dairy products. In untreated celiac disease, the small-intestinal enterocytes are severely damaged resulting in disaccharidase deficiency. This may cause persistent diarrhea and abdominal bloating if milk and dairy products are ingested. As the morphology of the mucosa improves, lactase activity tends to return to normal within a few months. In some cases, avoidance or reduction of lactose-containing products may be indicated for a short period after diagnosis before full-strength cow's milk and dairy products can be reintroduced in the diet. A few patients can never tolerate these foods and have to exclude them for life. Under these circumstances, dietary calcium intake will be reduced and it is wise to give supplements.

Restriction of other foods. Rarely, some patients only return to full health when foods such as eggs, chicken, tuna and soy are removed from the diet. Great care needs to be taken not to exclude foods to which patients may not, in fact, be sensitive. Restriction of dairy products and other foods must be carefully monitored, because compliance is often jeopardized as the diet becomes more limited.

111

Steroids. A few adult patients are ill at presentation and may benefit from a short course of steroids while the GFD is taking effect. Children never require steroids in this way.

If these simple steps are not effective or patients are giving particular concern, it may well be that the presence of a second diagnosis is responsible for clinical or histological non-response as already discussed (see pages 48–55). A number of these conditions are amenable to specific treatments that will improve or restore patients to full health. Those who have refractory celiac disease type 1 can often be treated successfully with steroids and azathioprine, but there are no proven satisfactory treatments for type 2 refractory celiac disease, which carries a poor prognosis.

Supplements. Patients are often deficient in iron, folic acid, calcium and vitamin D, and supplements should be given as required.

Response to treatment

After starting a GFD, symptomatic children show progressive clinical improvement and weight gain that parallel the healing of the celiac enteropathy. The first signs of amelioration are often seen within a few days, with increased appetite and mood change, but it may take some months before symptoms disappear completely. In typical cases, the response to treatment is sometimes prodigious, so that a severely malnourished and miserable child is rapidly transformed into a sturdy and healthy youngster.

Most adults also respond dramatically to a GFD, and the clinical and morphologic improvements usually occur in parallel, though clinical improvement can occur without normalization of the biopsy appearances. Healing of the small-intestinal lesion may require 1 or 2 years of treatment with a GFD. Anti-tissue transglutaminase (tTG) titer returns to normal usually within 6 to 24 months and this value can be used as an index of dietary compliance. Immunoglobulin (Ig)A anti-endomysial antibody (AEA) also disappears in those on a strict GFD. Abnormal IgG anti-gliadin antibody (AGA) levels may persist for longer, because of so-called immunologic memory. It should be noted that all the serological tests for celiac disease are too insensitive to detect minor transgressions of the diet.

Follow up

Patients should be followed up for life, preferably in a specialist clinic or by a family doctor with a particular interest in celiac disease, otherwise they are more likely to stray from the GFD. After diagnosis and the introduction of a GFD, patients should be reviewed after 3–6 months to ensure that they are making satisfactory progress and managing the diet. A follow-up intestinal biopsy is no longer recommended for confirmation of diagnosis. If all is well, patients should be reviewed annually, or sooner if problems arise. This is advisable in order that:

- any health concerns and associated disorders or complications that may have arisen can be addressed
- weight in adults, and growth and development in children, can be monitored
- blood tests can be carried out to monitor hematologic and biochemical indices, particularly hemoglobin, iron, folate and calcium
- adherence to the GFD can be assessed by dietary history and measurement of anti-tTG
- the need for other investigations, such as further small-bowel biopsies and scans for osteoporosis, can be assessed
- current membership of a celiac society can be confirmed.

Advice for celiac families

Parents with celiac disease, or other relatives with the condition, often ask whether their children are likely to develop the disorder. Celiac disease does run in families, but not in a predictable fashion. If the disorder is present in a family, the chance of another member being affected is about one in ten. Family members can now be screened easily with serological tests and small-intestinal biopsies should be carried out in those who are positive. Lack of HLA-DQ2 or -DQ8 virtually excludes the possibility of celiac disease developing in individuals with a family history.

When a new baby is born into a family with celiac disease, parents should be advised to introduce gluten at the same age as for any child (6–9 months). After this period, normal gluten intake should be achieved. It is important that babies are fed normally rather than given a low-gluten diet so that celiac disease, if present, will become evident. This will allow diagnosis and prompt treatment.

Role of celiac societies

At the time of diagnosis, all celiac patients should be advised to join the national celiac society and support one of the local groups in their area. These non-profit-making organizations, which are made up of and run by celiac patients and their families, fulfill a number of important functions by:

- helping patients to follow a GFD by producing comprehensive handbooks of the gluten-free foods that are available
- acting as a stimulus so that companies produce a wide range of palatable attractive foods
- encouraging hotels and restaurants to cater for celiac patients
- promoting meetings and producing videos, journals and other literature designed to inform patients about the condition
- raising the profile of celiac disease in the community
- raising funds for research into celiac disease.

Key points – management

- Treatment of celiac disease is based on the lifelong exclusion of wheat, rye and barley proteins from the diet.
- The intake of some nutrients tends to be lower than normal with the gluten-free diet (GFD), particularly fiber, iron, calcium and folates, and should be carefully monitored.
- Attention should be paid to avoid the ingestion of 'hidden' gluten (e.g. in sausages, cheese spreads, soups, soy sauce, mixed seasonings, malt beer and some medications and vitamin supplements).
- Gluten contamination of food that is suitable for celiacs (gluten threshold) should be kept as low as possible.
- The emotional and social implications of living without gluten on a lifelong basis should not be underestimated.
- Patients should be followed up for life, preferably in a specialist clinic, so that adherence to treatment can be monitored, nutritional and psychological advice can be given, and early diagnosis of possible complications can be made.

Key references

Catassi C, Fabiani E, Iacono G et al. A prospective, double blind, placebo-controlled trial to establish a safe gluten threshold for patients with celiac disease. *Am J Clin Nutr* 2007;85:160–6.

Ciacci C. The happy Scandinavian celiac world. *Dig Liver Dis* 2006;38: 181–2.

Haboubi NY, Taylor S, Jones S. Coeliac disease and oats: a systematic review. *Postgrad Med J* 2006;82: 672–8.

Hallert C, Svensson M, Tholstrup J, Hultberg B. Clinical trial: B vitamins improve health in patients with coeliac disease living on a gluten-free diet. *Aliment Pharmacol Ther* 2009;29:811–16.

Lee AR, Ng DL, Zivin J, Green PH Economic burden of a gluten-free diet. *J Hum Nutr Diet* 2007;20: 423–30.

Niewinski MM. Advances in celiac disease and gluten-free diet. *J Am Diet Assoc* 2008;108:661–72.

Roos S, Kärner A, Hallert C. Psychological well-being of adult coeliac patients treated for 10 years. *Dig Liver Dis* 2006;38:177–80.

Sverker A, Hensing G, Hallert C. 'Controlled by food' – lived experiences of coeliac disease. *J Hum Nutr Diet* 2005;18:171–80.

Troncone R, Auricchio R, Granata V. Issues related to gluten-free diet in coeliac disease. *Curr Opin Clin Nutr Metab Care* 2008;11:329–33.

Verbeek WHM, Schreurs MWJ, Visser OJ et al. Novel approaches in the management of refractory celiac disease. *Expert Rev Clin Immunol* 2008;4:205–19.

In recent years, concepts of celiac disease have undergone a revolution and have paved the way for further developments. With the advent of astonishingly sophisticated techniques in molecular medicine, advances in knowledge are assured and a new phase in the understanding of celiac disease is dawning.

Mechanisms causing mucosal damage

The most favored view is that the primary mechanism of mucosal damage is linked to the activation of T cells in the lamina propria by class II human leukocyte antigen (HLA)-restricted gliadin-presenting cells. This triggers a cascade of reactions leading to and sustaining mucosal damage. T-cell reactions in the adaptive immune response do not, however, explain the whole pathogenesis; the influence of other cells, such as macrophages and their cytokines, that contribute to the innate immune response is receiving increasing attention.

An intriguing question is why only some people develop celiac disease. In this regard attention is focusing on tissue transglutaminase, an enzyme that enhances the binding of gluten peptides to genetically determined heterodimers on antigen-presenting cells by a process of deamidation. This is a key step in the etiology of celiac disease. It may be that normally the enzyme is largely inactive and so not available to produce the crucial peptides that trigger particularly the adaptive immune response that leads to damage of the small-bowel mucosa. In celiac disease, the enzyme might be easily unmasked by, say, a bowel infection, excess gluten or other stresses and so starts the cascade of events leading to the celiac enteropathy. Even if some T cells are normally sensitized to gluten, these may be eliminated before they can release pro-inflammatory cytokines that would damage the mucosa, whereas in celiac disease these cells persist. So the role of tissue transglutaminase and the regulation of T cells in celiac disease would appear to be targets for research.

More detailed knowledge of the role of intestinal permeability, the trimolecular complex of the T-cell receptor, the HLA molecule and the damaging gliadin fragment will be forthcoming and will help not only to explain etiology and pathogenesis but also to develop new approaches to treatment. The development of an animal model would greatly accelerate progress.

Diagnosis

Diagnosis still rests on finding a characteristic enteropathy on histological examination of small-bowel biopsies. However, this is only one aspect of gluten sensitivity. Attention will focus on those patients with suspected celiac disease whose small-intestinal biopsies appear normal or near normal; such patients, in whom anti tissue transglutaminase antibody (anti-tTG) can be detected in the serum and who have evidence of gluten sensitivity, have already been described. Diagnosis is important because a gluten-free diet (GFD) restores health in those with symptoms and may prevent the future development of celiac disease with a severe enteropathy and all the attendant health risks.

Why some patients with gluten sensitivity have a normal biopsy while others have a severe enteropathy is unknown. It may be that distinct genetic factors regulate susceptibility to gluten sensitivity and enteropathy. It is likely that serological and genetic markers will define celiac disease more accurately in the future and so reduce the requirement for intestinal biopsy.

Awareness of celiac disease

Celiac disease is underdiagnosed. This is true not only for those with atypical presentations, but also for those with gastrointestinal complaints. This is unacceptable because there is a very effective treatment that not only restores patients to good health, but prevents complications. A greater awareness of the many ways that celiac disease may present is essential. This will be achieved by wide dissemination of information through medical journals, in the undergraduate medical curriculum, in postgraduate meetings, by manufacturers of gluten-free foods and by celiac societies. The increasing use of serological tests and endoscopic biopsy will uncover many more cases in the future.

The gluten-free diet

In recent years, the variety of gluten-free foods has increased enormously, mainly as a result of pressure from patients and their celiac societies. New ingredients for the GFD are currently under evaluation (e.g. sorghum), while new technologies (e.g. treatment of gluten-free bread with transglutaminase) are constantly improving the quality of food that is suitable for individuals with celiac disease. Food labeling, while improving, is still unsatisfactory. Patients can be unaware that certain foods contain gluten because of imprecise information on food labels. There are moves to remedy some of the difficulties, but pressure in this area needs to be maintained.

Treatments

Why an alternative to a gluten-free diet? The cornerstone of treatment of celiac disease is lifelong adherence to a strict GFD. However, gluten is a common and often unlabeled ingredient in the human diet, presenting a big challenge for patients. Gluten-free products are not widely available everywhere and are more expensive than their gluten-containing counterparts. Dietary compliance is therefore suboptimal in a large proportion of patients, particularly in developing countries. More than 50% of people that embrace a diet for medical reasons (e.g. hypertension, obesity, high cholesterol, diabetes and kidney failure) fail to comply over time, making any diet therapy a high-risk proposition. Furthermore, even when compliance is not an issue, a high percentage of patients with celiac disease on a GFD who are symptom free and test negative for serology show persistence of severe intestinal damage.

Potential new therapies: future without the gluten-free diet? The aforementioned progress made in understanding the cellular and molecular basis of celiac disease led to the identification of potential targets for therapy (Figure 10.1). At the time of writing, there are five active clinical trials registered at www.clinicaltrials.gov focused on alternative treatments to the GFD.

Enzyme therapy. The high proline content of gliadin peptides makes these molecules highly resistant to digestive processing by pancreatic and brush border proteases. Enzyme supplement therapy with prolyl

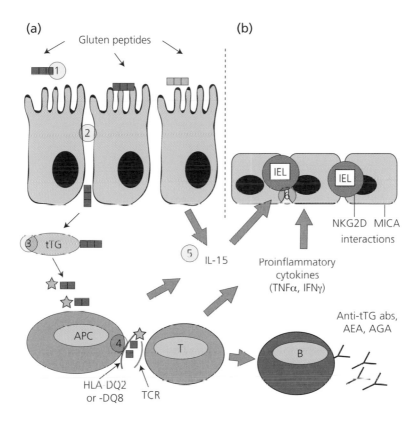

Figure 10.1 Targets for potential treatments of celiac disease other than the gluten-free diet in (a) normal mucosa and (b) celiac enteropathy. (1) Two trials are focusing on the use of prolyl endopeptidases to dismantle toxic gliadin peptides. (2) One trial is employing a zonulin inhibitor to correct the intestinal barrier defect typical of celiac disease. (3) Selective inhibition of tissue transglutaminase (tTG) in the small intestine may be a useful treatment. (4) The crucial role of the human leukocyte antigen (HLA) receptor makes it an obvious target for therapeutic intervention. (5) Antibodies to interleukin (IL)-15 have been proposed, particularly in the treatment of refractory celiac disease because of the intraepithelial lymphocyte (IEL)-activating role of IL-15. (6) A trial is in progress to evaluate the use of an inhibitor of the CCR-9 chemokine receptor that regulates homing of activated immune cells to the intestinal mucosa. AEA, anti-endomysial antibody; AGA, anti-gliadin antibody; IFN, interferon; TCR, T-cell receptor; TNF, tumor necrosis factor.

endopeptidases of different origin (bacterial, fungal or cereal-derived) has been proposed to promote complete digestion of cereal proteins and thus destroy T-cell multipotent epitopes. It remains to be assessed to what extent such intraluminal digestion may detoxify peptides particularly active in the most proximal part of the small intestine.

An alternative approach to reduce gluten toxicity is based on a pretreatment of whole gluten or gluten-containing food with bacterial-derived peptidase. Enzymatic detoxification of gluten has the potential to be an effective method for producing more palatable gluten-free products for treating celiac disease. Proteases of certain lactobacilli present in sourdough can proteolyze proline-rich gluten peptides. In a study, participants with celiac disease subjected to an acute challenge tolerated breads produced with sourdough (lactobacillus digested) better than those made with baker's yeast.

Engineered grains and inhibitory gliadin peptides. Breeding programs and/or transgenic technology may lead to production of wheat that is devoid of biologically active peptide sequences. Genetic engineering of non-toxic wheat that would not affect the baking properties has also been proposed, though the number and the repetition of such sequences in wheat render this approach challenging. The identification of specific epitopes may also provide a target for immunomodulation of antigenic peptides. According to the nature and position of the amino acid residues interacting with the specific T-cell receptor, peptide recognition can result in cellular activation (agonist), ignorance (null peptides) or unresponsiveness, known also as anergy (antagonist). Peptide analogs of gliadin epitope(s) can be engineered with antagonistic effects of native peptide(s). Of course, the chances of successfully using analog peptides to modulate specific immune responses could be hampered by the great heterogeneity of gliadin T-cell epitopes so far identified. Further studies to elucidate the hierarchy of pathogenic gliadin epitopes and their core region would be of crucial importance for engineering peptide-based therapy.

Immunomodulatory strategies. In the gut the autoantigenic enzyme tissue transglutaminase (tTG) is mainly expressed in the lamina propria and its expression is upregulated by various stimuli, such as mechanical stress, or bacterial or viral infection during a phase of active celiac disease. The enzyme catalyzes gluten deamidation and interaction with a glutamine-acceptor protein, increasing the rate of the protein's complex phagocytosis by antigen-presenting cells. Although the precise molecular details of this interaction in vivo remain unclear, selective inhibition of tTG in the small intestine might represent a therapeutically useful strategy for countering the immunotoxic response to dietary gluten in celiac disease. The substitution of a glutamine residue with 6-diazo-5-oxo-norleucine (DON) transforms an immunodominant gluten peptide into a potent inhibitor of tTG. DON-modified peptides could be useful for the study and therapy of celiac disease. However, the efficacy and side effects of tTG inhibitors are unknown.

The crucial role of the HLA receptor makes it an obvious target for therapeutic intervention. Furthermore, other immunomodulatory pathways, including interleukin (IL)-10, are possible alternative targets for promoting tolerance. However, evidence that gluten toxicity is not dependent only on T-cell recognition is growing. Activation of innate immunity has been demonstrated, and antibodies to IL-15 have been proposed, particularly in the treatment of refractory sprue because of the role of IL-15 in activating intraepithelial lymphocytes. Nevertheless, one should realize that treated celiac disease is a benign condition and dietary treatment is safe, although strenuous. Therefore, any immunomodulatory approach must have a safety profile equivalent to that of the GFD, but with the advantage of increased compliance.

Correction of the intestinal barrier defect. Small-intestinal permeability abnormalities are seen in patients with celiac disease (see Chapter 3). The use of the zonulin inhibitor AT1001 to correct intestinal barrier defects has been already successfully explored in an animal model of autoimmunity. More recently, AT1001 has been tested in an inpatient double-blind randomized placebo-controlled human clinical trial to determine its safety, tolerability and preliminary efficacy. No increase in adverse events was recorded among patients exposed to AT1001 compared with placebo. Following acute gluten exposure, a 70% increase in intestinal permeability was detected in the placebo group, while no changes were reported in the AT1001 group. After gluten exposure, interferon (IFN)γ levels increased in 4 out of 7 patients (57.1%) of the placebo group, but only in 4 out of 14 patients (28.6%)

of the AT1001 group. Gastrointestinal symptoms were significantly more frequent among patients in the placebo group than in those in the AT1001 group. Combined, these data suggest that AT1001 is well tolerated and appears to reduce gluten-induced intestinal barrier dysfunction, proinflammatory cytokine production and gastrointestinal symptoms in patients with celiac disease.

Primary prevention

Prevention is better than cure, and celiac disease may well be a preventable condition. It is caused by a complex interaction between genetic and environmental factors. Primary prevention of celiac disease is, therefore, theoretically possible by manipulating the environmental triggers that lead to the disorder in genetically predisposed individuals. Factors that appear to modulate the risk of the development of celiac disease include the pattern of infant feeding, early infection, the amount and quality of ingested gluten and the processes of fermentation of gluten-containing cereals. Analysis of an epidemic of early celiac disease in Sweden suggested that prolonged breastfeeding coupled with the introduction of small amounts of gluten while the infant is still being breastfed can reduce the risk of disease development. Infants initially exposed to cereals between the ages of 0 and 3 months or at 7 months or older have an increased risk of developing islet cell and/or celiac-type autoantibodies compared with those exposed during the fourth, fifth and sixth months. Prospective studies on infants at family risk of celiac disease are currently in progress to explore and extend these findings.

Epidemiology

Epidemiological studies of celiac disease continue to fascinate and raise intriguing questions. Why, for example, is celiac disease so rare among blacks – despite extensive years of experience, the British author of this book has never encountered a case. Presumably genetic factors are at work here. Studies now indicate an increasing prevalence of celiac disease that cannot be attributed solely to better detection rates. These aspects of celiac disease await further exploration and may shed light on the etiology of celiac disease itself.

And finally ...

Celiac disease is not only a common clinical problem, it is attracting worldwide research interest as never before from those working in a multitude of disciplines including clinical medicine, molecular medicine, pathology, genetics, biochemistry, immunology, epidemiology, pharmacology and food science. In the 1950s, when gluten was identified as the damaging agent and the discovery that a flat small-intestinal biopsy identified the disorder, researchers undoubtedly thought that finding the cause – an enzyme deficiency – lay just around the corner. Celiac disease has, however, been a hard nut to crack and while astonishing progress has been made in clarifying many aspects, particularly in the last 10 years, much remains tantalizingly elusive. The small bowel gives up its secrets slowly but who knows what the next decade will bring, with the amazing investigative tools available. But a word of caution, if the past is anything to go by, it may be many more years before the full story of this fascinating disorder can be told.

Key references

Branski D, Fasano A, Troncone R. Latest developments in the pathogenesis and treatment of celiac disease. *J Pediatr* 2006;149:295–300.

Di Cagno R, De Angelis M, Auricchio S et al. Sourdough bread made from wheat and nontoxic flours and started with selected lactobacilli is tolerated in celiac sprue patients. *Appl Environ Microbiol* 2004;70:1088–96.

Fasano A, Shea-Donohue T. Mechanisms of disease: the role of intestinal barrier function in the pathogenesis of gastrointestinal autoimmune diseases. *Nat Clin Pract Gastroenterol Hepatol* 2005;2: 416–22.

Sollid LM, Khosla C. Future therapeutic options for celiac disease. *Nat Clin Pract Gastroenterol Hepatol* 2005;2:140–7.

van Heel DA, West J. Recent advances in coeliac disease. *Gut* 2006;55:1037–46.

Useful resources

UK

British Society of Gastroenterology
3 St Andrews Place
Regent's Park
London NW1 4LB
Tel: +44 (0)20 7935 3150
www.bsg.org.uk

Coeliac Disease Resource Centre
Glutafin
Unit 3, Rowan House
Sheldon Business Park, Chippenham
Wiltshire SN14 0SQ
Professional helpline:
+44 (0)1249 466280
Glutafin consumer careline:
0800 988 2470
cdrc@glutafin.co.uk
www.cdrc.org.uk
Patient website: www.glutafin.co.uk

Coeliac UK
3rd Floor, Apollo Centre
Desborough Road
High Wycombe
Bucks HP11 2QW
Tel: +44 (0)1494 437 278
Helpline: 0870 444 8804
www.coeliac.org.uk

CORE (Digestive Disorders Foundation)
Freepost LON4268
London NW1 0YT
Tel: +44 (0)20 7486 0341
info@corecharity.org.uk
www.corecharity.org.uk

Primary Care Society for Gastroenterology
21 Tower Street
Covent Garden
London WC2H 9NS
Tel: +44 (0)20 7836 0088
secretariat@pcsg.org.uk
www.pcsg.org.uk

USA

American Celiac Disease Alliance
2504 Duxbury Place
Alexandria, VA 22308
Tel: +1 703 622 3331
info@americanceliac.org
www.americanceliac.org

American College of Gastroenterology
PO Box 342260
Bethesda, MD 20827–2260
Tel: +1 301 263 9000
www.acg.gi.org

American Gastroenterological
Association
4930 Del Ray Avenue
Bethesda, MD 20814
Tel: +1 301 654 2055
member@gastro.org
www.gastro.org

Celiac Disease Foundation
13251 Ventura Blvd 1
Studio City, CA 91604
Tel: +1 818 990 2354
cdf@celiac.org
www.celiac.org

Celiac Sprue Association
PO Box 31700
Omaha, NE 68131-0700
Tel: +1 402 558 0600
celiacs@csaceliacs.org
www.csaceliacs.org

National Foundation for Celiac
Awareness
PO Box 544
Ambler, PA 19002-0544
Tel: +1 215 325 1306
info@celiaccentral.org
www.celiaccentral.org

**International
Association of European Coeliac
Societies**
www.aoecs.org

Canadian Celiac Association
www.celiac.ca

The Coeliac Society of Australia
www.coeliacsociety.com.au

The Celiac Society of Italy
www.celiachia.it
www.celiachia.it/links/world.asp
(links to other national celiac societies)

European Society for Primary
Care Gastroenterology
www.espcg.org

United European
Gastroenterology Foundation
www.uegf.org

Further reading

Arendt EK, Dal Bello F, eds. *Gluten-free Cereal Products and Beverages. Food Science and Technology, International Series.* Academic Press, 2008.

Catassi C, Fasano A, Corazza GR, eds. *The Global Village of Celiac Disease. Perspective on Celiac Disease*, vol 2. Pisa: AIC Press, 2005.

Fasano A, Troncone R, Branski D, eds. *Frontiers in Celiac Disease. Pediatr Adolesc Med*, vol 12. Basel: Karger, 2008.

Mulder C, Cellier C, eds. *Coeliac Disease. Best Practice & Research Clinical Gastroenterology*, vol 12. Amsterdam: Elsevier, 2005.

Index